Inclusion Through Shared Education

Joanne Deppeler
Monash University, Australia

Danielle Zay
University of Charles de Gaulle Lille 3, France

Editors

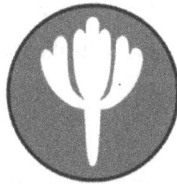

DEEP UNIVERSITY PRESS
Blue Mounds, Wisconsin

Deep University Online !

deepuniversitypress.org

For updates and more resources
Visit the Deep University Website:
www.deepuniversity.net
www.deepapproach.net

Certificate in Deep Education:
www.deepuniversity.net/graduatecourses.html

For permissions, contact: publisher@deepuniversity.net

ISBN   978-1-939755-29-2 (Paperback)

Library of Congress Cataloguing-in-Publication Data

1. Education and Society, Social Justice, Human Rights, Inclusion, Education, Special Education

Keywords: inclusive values, inclusive education, social justice, human rights, social actors, school and civil society, community partnership, shared responsibility

Target audience: Education and society courses, students and researchers in inclusive education, vocational education, special education, counsellors, speech therapists, parents

Deep University Press
Book Series "Inclusive Education and Partnerships"
Book Series editor: Danielle Zay

Table of contents

Acknowledgements

The introduction and chapters of this book were first published in French as a special issue, *Recherches & Educations,* 2015, October (14), review journal of the Binet-Simon Society (http://alfredbinet.univ-lorraine.fr/). The authors from the different countries represented in this volume participated in writing the editorial.

We thank Bernard Andrieu, professor, University of Paris Descartes (Sorbonne Paris City), President of the Binet-Simon Society and Editor-in-Chief of *Recherches & Educations* (http://recherches educations.revues.org) for allowing the special issue to be published in English.

This double publication in both French and English is an example of the strength of the international collaboration achieved between Deep University Press and the Binet-Simon Society and its review. This publication is a timely introduction to the 2017 Binet-Simon Society international Conference, to be held in Paris. The conference will celebrate the one hundred sixtieth anniversary of Alfred Binet's birth. Binet's archives were inherited and are published by the Binet-Simon Society. Alfred Binet was a trailblazer, well ahead of his time in his thinking about psychology and education. He could be considered as a trailblazer in the field of inclusive education.

In the USA, Isabelle Druc translated the introduction to the book for the back cover and formatted the whole for Deep University Press, while Janine Kam reviewed some of the English texts. We also benefited from the advice of François V. Tochon, University of Wisconsin-Madison. Thank you to them.

Joanne Deppeler, Professor and Associate Dean of Graduate Research in the Faculty of Education, Monash University, Australia

Danielle Zay, Professor Emeritus, University of Charles de Gaulle Lille 3, France. Book Series Editor "Inclusive Education and Partnerships", Deep University Press.

Introduction
Inclusive Education Through Shared Education

Joanne Deppeler
Monash University, Australia

Danielle Zay
University of Charles de Gaulle Lille 3, France

In a democracy, education is viewed as the primary mechanism through which opportunities exist for everyone to succeed and to build a prosperous future, irrespective of their personal or social circumstances. To what extent are the benefits of educational success available to all in modern democracies? What is meant by inclusive education? How might we recognise and accommodate the multitude of definitions and the resulting confusion of interpretation of the concept of inclusive education? International agreements and legislation provide definitions of inclusive education that focus on equity, access, opportunity and rights as the basis for education policy and the foundation for a just society. The lack of an agreed conceptual frame for inclusive education may contribute to its misconception and confused practice (Forlin et al., 2013). So much research has been published in this area that it would be futile to attempt to undertake a comprehensive summary of the field.

The primary purpose of this issue is more modest. In attempting to address these questions, we bring together authors from the West to the East, including Canada, USA, France, Great Britain, Spain,

Australia, China, Taiwan, and who represent a range of cultures around the theme of *Inclusion through shared education*. Each case provides a snapshot of inclusion by sharing values, ideas, knowledge, educational work among various partners, in and out of school and/or in terms of research and writing.

Two main directions can be identified in the evolution of inclusive education. The first emanates from those organisations which deal with the problems of disabled persons with a view to allowing them not to be discriminated against in relation to other people in society or at school. Then, this was broadened to include all young people having difficulties at school and allocated to classes or pathways, which did not allow them to participate in inclusive education.

In both of these cases, there is the clear affirmation of the right of every human being to education and the study of the approaches and practices that are likely to reform education systems in ways that provide positive environments that retain all students.

The first two chapters, those of Danielle Zay (France) and Lena de Botton and other contributors of the INCLUD-ED team under the direction of Ramon Flecha (University of Barcelona, Spain), are situated within the broader perspective of concurrent transformations and the interaction between school and society, in funded research supported by various European programs focused on such links.

Zay analyses the development of the concept of inclusive education drawing from the movement for human rights and the theory of justice by Rawls (1999), revisited by Sen (2009). In view of the latter, a proper respect for the rights of every human being can be built only through dialogue and negotiation between social actors, since each context is unique and no universal theory of justice can resolve disputes it raises. In education, this implies a constructivist approach to guide cognitive acquisitions in the same way that knowledge develops scientifically, through formulating and testing hypotheses that may be proven false, and through discussing different points of view on the matter, those of experts, practitioners, users and of who-do-not-know but think they know.

In a society where everyone is exposed to a flotilla of information, the role of the school is not so much to import ready-made content but to analyse what content is delivered and to know how to 'triage/sort through' what is relevant and what is not. Such an approach is part of citizenship education, because it implies listening to others, respecting their ideas, and resolving conflicts through well thought-out discourse and not through either symbolic or physical force (Moje, 2007; Zay, 2012). The chapter concludes with a questioning of the role of civil society, and especially, the role of groupings, in order to change society and school at the same time.

Lena de Botton and her colleagues discuss the case study of a school in Spain which was about to close and which has been transformed by mobilizing existing human resources in the surrounding community to support learning. "Interactive groups" were formed with heterogeneous students in terms of their level of performance in the field, gender, culture and ethnicity. The adults supervising the students came from varied backgrounds, i.e. students, community volunteers, family members, former students and other people from the surrounding area. The diversity of interactions was an advantage that helped to break down social stereotypes. Often, basic training was needed for the families. Relationships with knowledge grow in the families. The degree of improvement in school academic performance improvement results demonstrated that the approach is proving to be effective.

Eighty-five percent of women obtained employment after the school year in the local district or nearby region. This outcome was made possible by the training and the accomplishments achieved through the work. Neighbours became involved in the administration outside of the school, creating spaces for dialogue joint committee meetings or at school, formulating effective solutions for the community. This chapter presents the advantages of a local education policy, which relies on its social environment. It is based on the results of research in a Spanish primary school, but its scope goes well beyond the case study presented. Indeed, the transferability of the results has been studied in six European educational centres.

In contrast, the Australian team consisting of members from different countries under the direction of Joanne Deppeler analyse the challenges faced by the education system of a country divided between states and territories, and which is moving towards a strengthening of federal policy to ensure a more equitable the rights for students with disabilities. Indeed, numerous issues appear to arise from the disparate nature and types of services offered and the lack of consistency in the reporting of outcomes from alternative curricula, which often do not provide sufficient information. "The lack of consistency means it is difficult to determine whether appropriate progress is being made by students with varying levels of disability" which in turns hinders decision making in relation to national and regional examinations and the future planning which should flow from these. No legal obligation exists to enable schools to put into place alternative tests adapted to the different levels of disability. Standards of educational accountability for students with a disability appear substantially less than for the regular student cohort, as many students do not seem to participate in national testing. It is argued that if Australia is to overcome the current inequities in provision and better understand how diversity and disadvantage might be addressed collaboration among families, educators and health professionals and engagement with politicians will be required to achieve the goals of fairness and inclusive education.

The chapters about a Spanish village and the Australian states and territories are in line with different inclusive education policies, one based on local action, the other to correct the effects of it through national practices. In both cases, the authors argue that successful implementation of such a policy requires shared design in education. The first case advocates links with the authorities in the school context, which forms the environment in which the learning is developing. In the second case, emphasis is placed on direct links between established institutions, special and regular schools and collaboration among families and professionals and university-school partnerships in order to support a more inclusive education system overall. Thus, any step bringing together most of the social players involved with education has possibilities for finding better solutions (Deppeler, 2014). Ultimately, the authors agree with Zay's conclusion, a process for inclusive education involves not only educators, but dialogue amongst these, other citizens and politicians in order to proceed in the direction of both pedagogical reforms and fairer social changes, each one being linked to the designs and values of everyone.

With the next three chapters, we leave the influence of policy on educational practices, to focus on the experiences of people with disabilities and to those who welcome them and accompany them in the education system.

François V. Tochon (USA) and Yi-hung Liao (Taiwan) analyse and attempt to make sense of the lived experiences of disability and impairment. They respond to similar questions posed by the study of Australian policy and practice, investigating both the progress in alternative spaces, also the potential of those which could be created. Their research clarifies the way in which the identity of a person with a disability is produced. Two hypotheses underlie the debate. On the one hand, identity and subjectivity are often interchangeable, subjectivity having "a reflexive property (one's own sense of self) which is continually reconstructed in and through discourse. On the other hand, the identity emerges from discourse interactions in the play of power relations that normalize and regulate the body and the discourses responsible for identity formation.

From Foucault's (2003) genealogical method, the study of life stories of hearing impaired students in foreign language classes in the first year of university in Taiwan brings to light how discursive practices which form learning experiences are influenced by power relationships. The terms used by the students bring to light the way in which a view of difference in a sense of identity transforms this view into a feeling of inferiority in respect of a world dominated by normal people. It would constitute "an invisible eugenic process".

The Quebec team, Corina Borri-Anadon et al., delve more deeply into this issue through interviews with school speech therapists managing students from ethnic, cultural, and linguistic diversity who qualify for support because of their disability. The taking into account of the problem falls within a simplistic policy designed only in terms of the organization of educational services that promote the schooling of students struggling in so-called normal classes. The research analyses the double handicap faced by those considered as both deficient because of their personal characteristics classified from a psycho-medical perspective and from their connection to difference. The real-life situations are not perceived as being able to offer positive benefits, on the contrary, they weaken access to success.

In the argument around differentiation/standardisation/normalis- ation, differentiation and standardisation become two sides of the same reality of normalisation. Whether it is the recognition of impairment of the individual or the role of sociocultural factors in the individual's schooling, which predominate, the problem is situated in the student's body from the start or is aggravated by his/her environment. Inclusive principles affirmed in the discourse of speech therapists are at variance with the assessment practices, but the latter are influenced by organisational, material, or financial obstacles.

Claire de Saint Martin finds the same psycho-medical influences in French schools where orienting the diagnosis of the student's difficulties in relation to a "typology of deficiencies" was adopted in order to place him/her in a special class. This, in turn, hindered the possibility of valuing other personal or family and social conditions likely to favour access to academic success.

Within the context of socio-clinical institutional analysis (Monceau, 2003), the method involves subjects as a group leading them to exercise introspective skills and an elaboration of thought, which produces usable data. The students have differentiated discourse across their experience of inclusion, causing a process to emerge in different phases. At the beginning of a school with similar children in a special class, the students are happy because they are not aware of their differences. It is only when they are in a "normal class" and when the naming of these differences is reinforced by the visibility of their difficulties that they are disappointed. Immersion in the normal school environment remains partial. The student, after a process, which goes across years, can succeed in adapting to scholastic standards, but remains isolated and does not form connections with others except for those who are similar. Socialisation is a failure.

The six chapters use the term 'inclusive education" to describe systemic approach to education that involves complex interactions of factors, both within the educational system as an integral part of the society where the voting citizens have specific values and ideologies in each country. The chapters highlight the barriers impeding the generalisation of inclusive education. This goes well beyond the boundaries of national states with regard to a neo-liberal ideology, centred on the profit motive and competition favouring an approach to education that reduce the acquisition of skills and that are driven by the market (Deppeler et al. this volume).

Is the example of the Spanish community's collaborative efforts in transforming and preventing closure of their school, unique? (Botton, et al., this volume). Is inclusive education doomed to remain the result of local or regional initiatives that fail to generalise across the wider education system (Zay, 2012)?

References

Deppeler, J. (2014) Developing equitable practices in schools: professional collaboration in research. In Jones, P. (Ed.), *Bringing insider perspectives into inclusive teacher learning: Potentials and challenges for educational professionals* (178-188). New-York, NY: Routledge.

Forlin, C., Chambers, D., Loreman, T., Deppeler, J. M. & Sharma, U. (2013). *Inclusive education for students with disability: A review of the best evidence in relation to theory and practice, prepared for the Australian Government Department of Education, Employment and Workplace Relations.* Canberra, ACT: Australian Research Alliance for Children & Youth (ARACY). http://www.aracy.org.au/publications-resources/area?command=record&id=186

Foucault, M. (2003). *"Society must be defended": lectures at the College de France, 1975-76* (M. Bertani & A. Fontana Eds. D. Macey Trans.). New York: Picador.

Moje, E. B. (2007). Developing socially just subject-matter instruction: a review of the literature on disciplinary literacy teaching. *Review of Research in Education*, 31, 1-44.

Monceau, G. (2003). Pratiques socianalytiques et socio-clinique institutionnelle. *L'homme et la société*, 1, 147, 11-33.

Rawls, J. (1999). *A theory of justice.* Cambridge (Massachusetts): The Belknap Press of Harvard University Press, 1st ed. 1971.

Sen, A. (2009). *The idea of justice.* Cambridge (Massachusetts): The Belknap Press of Harvard University Press, 1st ed. 2009.

Zay, D. (2012). *L'éducation inclusive. Une réponse à l'échec scolaire?* Préface de Gabriel Langouët. Paris: Ed. L'Harmattan.

1

Inclusive Education and Social Change

Danielle Zay
University of Charles de Gaulle Lille 3, France

Abstract

Recent theoretical trends have prompted a rethinking of the concept of inclusive education to answer growing contestations from researchers and practitioners. This paper introduces a new interpretation of previous comparative research findings supported by European funding. The topic is no longer only pedagogical. Indeed, recent evolutions of Western democracies call for re-analysing the school system's underlying values as far as they are connected and interdependent of the society. Does the issue of achieving inclusive education highlight that there is a contradiction between the declared values of democratic societies and their ways of working? Are the latter generated by social forces, which oppose one another and thus build a society more or less based on exclusion? This paper analyses how oppositional values evident in schooling bring into question the role of civil society and social agents relative to the state in a globalized world.

Following the decision voted by the European Parliament in February 2014 to bring the national accounts of member states into line with the European System of Accounts (ESA 2010), a revised ESA came into effect in September 2014. The revised ESA included prostitution, drug trafficking and smuggled goods for the purposes of calculating their GDP (Gross Domestic Product). Indeed, this had previously been actioned in one form or another, in Belgium, Finland, Great-Britain, Italy, Norway, the Netherlands, Slovenia and Sweden (Rossi, 2014). The ESA revision allows increasing the GDP without changing anything else. On the one hand, nothing more is produced. On the other hand, austerity policies reducing social expenses for all citizens are maintained while inequalities and social exclusion caused by unemployment and poverty are increasing.

Is the revised GDP consistent with the EU (European Union) educational policy that endeavours to support and foster educational and social inclusion? In other words is this consistent with the goal to educate young people for democratic citizenship and respect for each other?

This chapter brings previous comparative education research findings into question by using a theoretical framework in which the concept of inclusion appears to be both confused and under threat (Allan, 2003), a "slogan" misused by politicians and that raises indignation from researchers and teacher unions (Thomas & Vaughan, 2009). Through the "readings and reflections" of the latter, it appears that the concept of inclusive education is rooted in various, intricate and intermingled conceptual, ideological and social networks. Inclusive education must therefore be reviewed on more than a single academic frame or methodology and include multiple approaches and research papers in order to highlight the evolution and changes in conceptual meanings through their heterogeneous applications and theoretical rebuilding.

The key question addressed in previous research remains: How can schools in isolation respond effectively to challenges that result from poverty and other social disadvantages without the combined support and effort of the wider society (Zay, 2005a, 2012a&b)? What is the impact of the various and often competing social forces and their ways of working on schools in a democracy?

A challenge in applying the principles of inclusive education is that they do not necessarily reveal the contradictions that exist between the democratic values espoused by society and the various oppositional ways of working that are enacted. Langouët (2014) used a set of data (income, health and education) collected by the (United Nations Development Program (UNDP) and compared the HDI (Human Development Index) to the GDP. The index adjusted by the Nobel Prize in Economics Amartya Sen took into account various factors of well-being of the population such as health and life expectancy, education, and work and leisure time (UNDP, United Nations Development Program, 2006). The basic criterion for measuring positive economic evolution was no longer focused only on the increase of goods, but on how they were distributed among all citizens and how they improve the quality of life for all.

In the following section, the evolution of the concept of inclusive education is discussed taking into account differences in definitions linked with principles of social justice. It is argued that this brings into question how a democratic society through schooling is able to resolve the conflicting values and the social forces that support these values in order to achieve its aim to be inclusive.

Towards making extensive meaning and use of inclusive education

The concept of inclusive education is increasingly used and misused in social and educational fields in a push towards "good practices" (Muskens, 2009, Zay, 2012a) based on measures of effectiveness (Loreman et al., 2014) [1]. This in turn puts inclusive education at risk for failure as a policy (Allan, 2003). Practitioners as well as researchers have attempted to analyse how this concept has been applied in several contexts and to clarify its various meanings. What is also questioned is whether the idea of inclusive education is in itself able to inspire social and educational changes towards a better democratic society.

To Allan (2003, p.1) "the purpose of inclusive education" is the same for all those involved in it, "teachers, teacher educators or researchers". Though she maintains focus on children with disabilities, she notes that inclusive education aims "to maximise the participation of young people in mainstream schools". She refers to several researchers to define inclusive education as "a complex process" that is jeopardised by "the regime of accountability" imposed by educational policies, including those entitled "inclusive". The "obsession of standards", delivered by "market ideologies" "eliminates democratic discussion about the purpose of schooling", and makes educational authorities reject the views of students and parents. Teacher education "reduces inclusion to a contrived cultural performance by professionals". In such conditions, increasing the number of children present in main schools is inefficient. Allan (2008, p.2) in referring to Derrida (1990), states "the desire for certainty within education" "creates closure in practices and profound injustices for particular individuals", and, "for instance about what constitutes good practice», «allows for the evasion of responsibility". In considering that the diversity of meanings, policies and practices inside and between countries Allan takes account of the "voices" and stories from young people, parents and professionals to coin her own definition of inclusive education. Allan (2008, p.226) concludes that we need to abandon the "narrow sense of inclusion that prevails nowadays" and consider the mutual goals of both inclusive education and democracy. The enduring challenge is to identify what forms of participation are necessary to achieve these goals.

Thomas and Vaughan (2009) elaborate the concept of inclusive education by analysing its changes of meaning through "the context – rights, participation, social justice", "the arguments and evidence against segregation – 1960s to day", "Legislation, reports, statements" (titles of their chapters).

Their work has inspired the present analysis of inclusive education that deepens their key idea: as soon as it emerges as in its different variations, the concept of inclusive education is underlain by recognizing equal rights to all human beings, whatever their different capacities are [2].

It is supported by values focusing on the significance of what the institutions, schools and others generate for those who depend on them. It is why the authors argue that a reference to Goffman goes to the heart of the topic

"not because it has anything specially to say about special education, but because in 1968 it marked the beginnings of a questioning of the automatic assumption that separation of a portion of the public to segregated institutions must be a good thing (…) These include mental hospitals, boarding schools and so on " (Thomas & Vaughan, 2009, p.31).

What is common with the present paper is the idea that such institutions "are constructed to serve the purpose of the wider system rather than the inhabitants of the institution" (ibid.).

In the same lineage of ideas, the authors date the emergence of the concept of inclusive education itself back to critics in the area of young disabled students and quote, in particular, the paper by Dunn (1968) entitled "Special education for the mildly retarded - is much of it justifiable?"

Thus, the concept of inclusive education appears to represent a confluence of several political, educational and social streams of thought. Its definition was renewed and strengthened by the call for social justice and its interpretation by researchers. In the 20th century, the most ancient call for human rights started again with de-segregation. King's (1992) "I have a dream" speech before the Lincoln memorial was a turning point of the civil rights movement in the sixties, in a country overwhelmed by a White majority. *The Theory of Justice* published by Rawls (1999) in 1971, then questioned and reinterpreted by Sen (2009), elaborated the theoretical background to allow a universal meaning of a social justice based on an inclusive society and its education system.

Introducing the notion of conceptual evolution may be questioned, because as Sen claims that there cannot be a "theory" but an "idea" of justice that is different for each of us. Therefore, it has to be negotiated in each specific context by those who need to make the decision. In contrast with a "theory" elaborated by a researcher using a top to bottom approach, such experiences can empower each individual, and build shared ideas of justice based on individuals feelings and perceptions. Thus the concept of justice becomes deeply rooted in the field and includes more and more citizens from bottom to top as a solid basis for a democratic society.

International institutions have articulated the ideas promoted by educational, social and theoretical circles making inclusive education an aim for policy for all countries claiming to be democratic.

While modifying regular schools for students with disabilities remains a focus, the concept aims to take into account discrimination and disadvantage of every kind, not only those due to individual factors (biological or psychological), but social, cultural, ethnic, and so on. Thus "Education for All", requires change to the whole educational system in order to best develop the potential of all young people.

Some significant turning points can be highlighted.

In 1989, *The U.N. Convention on the Rights of the Child (UNCR)* acknowledges in its title that it does not focus on the notion of need, but on the right of every human being (i.e. alone endowed with reason). Two centuries later, it acknowledges for children what was available for men at the Age of Kant, the Enlightenment philosophy and the Declaration of Human Rights of 1789. To Thomas & Vaughan (2009, p.3), referring to Hevey (1992), such a claim "calls for rights rather than charity". In other words, justice replaces acts of kindness.

Article 29 on the "Aims of education," expresses that the educational development of the individual is the central aim and that education should allow children to reach their fullest potential in terms of cognitive, emotional and creative capacities (UNESCO, 2005, p.12).

In 1994, the UNESCO (United Nations Educational, Scientific and Cultural Organization) re-enacts the UN Convention to make inclusion one of the Human and Child rights by making it ratified by representatives of 92 governments and 25 international organizations in *The Salamanca Statement and Framework for Action on Special Needs Education*. Thus it turns the issue terms round. As Lindqvist, the UN-Rapporteur, says:

> *"All children and young people of the world, with their individual strengths and weaknesses, with their hopes and expectations, have the right to education. It is not our education systems that have a right to certain types of children. Therefore, it is the school system of a country that must be adjusted to meet the needs of all children" (UNESCO, 2005, p.13).*

All governments are enjoined to make inclusion the lawful norm of the school system.

> *"The Conference proclaimed that: 'regular schools with [an] inclusive orientation are the most effective means of combating discriminatory attitudes, creating welcoming communities, building an inclusive society and achieving education for all; moreover, they provide an effective education to the majority of children and improve the efficiency and ultimately the cost-effectiveness of the entire education system' " (p. ix) (UNESCO, 2005, p.13).*

Subsequently, the UNESCO has never ceased from recommending this form of inclusive education. It has done this in two ways.

1. UNESCO highlighted that most educational needs don't come from students' inherent differences, but rather from the social conditions of their lives that create the consequent disadvantages in their education.

The World Education Forum meeting in Dakar, April 2000, listed them:

> *"the needs of the poor and the disadvantaged, including working children, remote rural dwellers and nomads, ethnic and linguistic minorities, children, young people and adults affected by conflict, HIV and AIDS, hunger and poor health, and those with disabilities or special learning needs. It emphasized the special focus on girls and women" (UNESCO, 2009, p.8).*

2. UNESCO (2005, p.13&15) differentiated inclusive education from being conceived to answer "special" needs of disabled students, to:

"a process of addressing and responding to the diversity of needs of all learners through increasing participation in learning, cultures and communities, and reducing exclusion within and from education [...] Inclusion is concerned with providing appropriate responses to the broad spectrum of learning needs in formal and non-formal educational settings. Rather than being a marginal issue on how some learners can be integrated in mainstream education, inclusive education is an approach that looks into how to transform education systems and other learning environments in order to respond to the diversity of learners. It aims towards enabling teachers and learners both to feel comfortable with diversity and to see it as a challenge and enrichment of the learning environment, rather than a problem."

The key word is diversity. Thus, the inclusive education raises an issue that is the same for both education and society: How do we live together with our differences? How do we ensure respect for including all equitably?

From inclusive education to putting society at stake through school

Since its emergence, whether focusing on an individual student with disabilities or on the school as a whole, the idea of inclusive education has drawn attention to the injustice caused to some who by virtue of their human nature should be endowed with the same rights as others. In attempting to analyse how school failure might be solved researchers have highlighted the entangled and complex situations of injustice in schooling and in the wider society.

The DOCA European documentary research analyses different kinds of remediation for students considered 'at risk' for school failure [3]. When the starting point for identifying pedagogical solutions arises from analysing "special needs", it can result in exclusion of young people considered "different" from their same age peers. This approach tends to increase the cases of difference: mentally, physically, linguistically, socially, culturally "handicapped" students. Such choices may legitimate an easy solution for teachers by shifting all of the trouble makers, as well as all those who slow down the learning pace, out of the regular classrooms. As a result, more and more students are pushed out of ordinary classrooms, schools, as the school system moves toward extensive segregation for the "poorly adapted".

Research and assessments highlight that segregated ways of remedying school failure are more or less successful as soon as the student is inside, but fail to achieve their final aim, making him/her successful when coming back to the compulsory schooling with his/her peers at the same age. The pupil has changed, but, if the school system remains the same, the same causes bring about the same effects. Dusseau and Isambert (2003, p.99), two French Chief Inspectors of Schools in charge of evaluating the class and rebound programmes, consider the return to mainstream school the ultimate aim of the rebound programme, as the "programmes' stumbling block». They consider more useful to prevent problems as soon as they occurred in a regular classroom.

In the ten countries investigated in the DOCA research, several successful factors appear (Muskens, 2009; Zay, 2012a&b). The main one, and the only one that is the same in all countries, is school staff motivation. Dusseau and Isambert (2003, p.32) also conclude about the same cause of their "positive assessment of diverse situations". To them too, it seems to be that "the commitment of the Heads of schools, teachers, teachers of children with special needs often come with their firm belief and a true militancy" (pp.163-164).

The same factors may be found in examples accounting for experiences in the field. For instance, in France on the website entitled "Le Café pédagogique" [4], with some outstanding landmarks such as "Le Forum des enseignants novateurs" (the Innovative Teachers' Forum), or, in the United Kingdom (UK), on "Schools Improvement Net " [5] as well as on TES (think, educate, share) [6].

To Schleicher, Director, Directorate for Education and Skills at the OECD (Organisation for Economic Co-operation and Development), PISA (Programme for International Student Assessment) results and their evolution since 2003 until 2012 show that "principals' and teachers' perception of disadvantage correlates with inequalities in education opportunities more strongly than real disadvantage does" (cf. OECD, 2013). It is why in PISA Top-performer Singapore, disadvantage is significant, but its impact on learning outcomes is only moderate. In contrast, France has less disadvantaged students, but school principals perceive it to be large, and student learning outcomes are closely related to social background [7].

The OECD (2010) highlights that education doesn't depend on educational staff' perceptions and motivations only, but that the whole social actors are doing it as it is: parents who educate their children and weigh on schools' staff decisions, citizens who elect representatives choosing educational policy, and so on.

> *"In the most successful education systems, the political and social leaders have persuaded their citizens to make the choices needed to show that they value education more than other things. But placing a high value on education will get a country only so far if the teachers, parents and citizens of that country believe that only some subset of the nation's children can or need to achieve world class standards. This report shows clearly that education systems built around the belief that students have different pre-ordained professional destinies to be met with different expectations in different school types tend to be fraught with large social disparities. In contrast, the best-performing education systems embrace the diversity in students' capacities, interests and social background with individualised approaches to learning"* (OECD, 2010, p.4).

French bad ranking comes from a more important number of students failing than in other countries, because social inequalities weigh on school success more than elsewhere. Indeed they are supported by elitist national features and a specific perception of education based on the value of "excellence". Excellence could be conceived as managing the most successful school system for all students, in other words, an inclusive education. But excellence, here, is conceived as selecting students to making some of them better than others that are considered as unable to do the best. This defines an exclusive education characterised by:

- a pedagogy based upon a way of teaching that focuses more on the subject matter than on the student learning;

- a teacher education that focuses more on academic graduates than on pedagogical skills and despises teacher training.

> *"(...) In France, 90% of teachers deem themselves well prepared or very well prepared with regard to the content of the subject they teach (cf. TALIS average of 93%). In contrast, nearly 40% of teachers feel inadequately prepared for the pedagogical aspects of teaching, which is the highest proportion in any of the 34 countries taking part in the TALIS survey"* (OECD 2014, p.5) [8].

There is a similar inedaquacy in the ongoing training available as in the school system. It is inadequately focused on the needs of the teachers, the proportion of teachers reported having undertaken a professional development activity over the past 12 months is lower than the average of survey countries and the training courses on offer to teachers are less intensive. "For example, the number of days spent by French teachers in courses or workshops is only half the average for TALIS survey countries" (ibid).

- In 2011, like most European countries, France invests over 6% of its GDP in education, but with a split between primary and secondary education. The French average salaries in pre-primary and primary education is respectively 7% and 17% below average for the OECD countries, but is " virtually equal " for secondary education (p.6). Per student on secondary education, France spends 20% more than the OECD average, but is 20% below the OECD average on primary (p.8). Yet, early education is the school level that allows socio-economically disadvantaged pupils to get some of the cultural level acquired by more advantaged pupils from their families before going to school, and not to remain too disadvantaged in the following levels.

- And to crown it all, a typical French educational system organization from the end of secondary to the higher education promotes the elites: the "classes préparatoires" located in upper secondary best "lycées", but after the "Baccalauréat (bac.)", secondary school leaving examination certificate taken at the end of secondary school. These preparatory classes train high-flying students for the competitive entrance exam for the "grandes écoles", that are higher education public or private institutions for civil servant students, like future teachers, or for CEO (Chief executive officers) of public or private firms and upper administration, or high qualified engineers. On the contrary, universities are obliged to accept all students who have passed the "bac". The conception of excellence is based on the greater number of candidates who fail. Thus the secondary schooling is influenced by raising the academic qualifications because of the need to prepare students to take a selective exam, even if most of them will not. The "grandes écoles" called "ENS" (Ecoles normales supérieures) prepare most of the successful candidates graduated as "agrégés". Only teachers who pass the "agrégation" can teach in preparatory classes. Whatever be the level of secondary education, they have higher salaries than other secondary teachers graduated as "certifiés" (OECD 2014, p.6) for less working hours.

Van Zanten & Maxwell (2015) analyze how the French very conservative and unequal educational system works being both negotiated between the state and the dominant social classes, and seen as a public good. Not only *A State Nobility* is remaining, like Bourdieu (1996) described it, but interpenetration between elites of state administration and business due to a closed education in preparatory classes and "grandes écoles" and the trust all upper circles in public and private firms have in such an education. Van Zanten & Maxwell (2015, p.79) quote studies showing that "a significant proportion of CEOs of the 40 largest French private firms are graduates from public grandes écoles" and that "among the 200 most important French companies, 47% in the 1980s and 28% in 2007 had among their directors people who had had a previous career in the public sector".

The authors argue that the educational policy to open the "grandes écoles" was successful for best students only to strengthen the elites. Padoani-David case study quoted in a chapter of Zay (2012a) analysed this policy from inside a business school in her Ph.D research. The initiative of welcoming the best students of upper secondary schools located in socio-economically deprived areas came from the IEP (Institut d'Etudes Politiques/Institute of Political Studies), "Sciences Po." (Political Sciences) Paris. In 2002, it was followed by one of the most renown business school, ESSEC (Ecole supérieure de Sciences économiques et commerciales/Economic and business sciences School), and institutionalised by a law in 2005. This specific policy of "equity of opportunities"- only for the best students of lower classes - is considered to be in the scope of the traditional Republican "meritocratic" system. But Padoani David shows that the "grandes écoles" needed to recruit students from a larger basis of recruitment to get the best and face the tough competition between them. The business and managerial schools promote very efficient pedagogical methods and devices, but these are not extended to the whole school system and are kept for a few.

These analyses incite to deepen the role played by values underlying social perceptions of school and society. The empirical research results of the British-French Interreg project encourage going further (Zay, 2005a, 2012b) [9].

Conflicting values and social forces in democracies aiming at inclusion

The comparative analyses of schools' local strategies when applying inclusive policies in France and England deepen the study of antagonistic models of society and school. They are supported by social forces managing to impose different ways of working in such and such sector of the former and the latter depending of their more or less strong influence on one or the other. This last part of the chapter, like the previous ones, tries to extend the interpretation of these research results. It does it by defining inclusive education as based on "the idea of justice". The issue leads to question the role played by social actors for maintaining or changing established situations that make most people disadvantaged.

The Interreg research data analyses were inspired by hypotheses suggested by Cousins (1998; Zay, 2005a&b, 2012b). From reviewing contemporary debates, she elaborated four European paradigms underlying conceptions of social justice and relationships between the individual and the society in each country. All the paradigms apply in all countries, but one of them prevails in each one. On one opposite side, in the Anglo-American specialisation paradigm underpinned by a neo-liberal overview of the world, social order depends on voluntary exchanges between autonomous individuals motivated by their own interests and each is responsible for his or her situation. All sectors of society, including school, depend on a self-regulating market and free competition including education. On the most opposite side, in the French solidarity paradigm, based upon the Durkheimian concept, the notion of social exclusion reflects a lack of solidarity as a rupture to the social fabric. The concept of republican citizenship gives rights and duties to all and an obligation for the state to help the excluded to be included. It inspires French welfare policy and, for instance, a measure such as the RMI (Revenu Minimal d'Insertion), that is to say minimum income for social integration. The problem is not only poverty, the lack of resources, but the lack of social participation that is to say to be deprived from the citizen's rights. In the same way, a supposedly strong administration is expected to operate regulation in order to guarantee equal opportunities for all (Zay, 2005a&b, 2012b).

After emerging in France in 1974, the concept of social exclusion spreaded to other European countries and institutions. The European Commission used it instead of poverty and set up the European Observatory on National Policies for Combating Social Exclusion in 1990.

Like paradigms of social exclusion,

"school models are in competition, and each one may struggle successfully in some part of the system relative to the strength of the competitive social forces which support them" (Zay, 2005a, p.110).

Lorcerie (1994) distinguishes three main competing school models in France since the eighties-nineties. In 1989, the Law of Orientation in Education clarified the opposition. Focusing on student's learning, "the core of the system", it made the Republican school focusing on teaching subject matter a first previous historical model. But Célestin Freinet in France, Ovide Decroly in Belgium or Maria Montessori in Italy already had advocated this "pedagogical" model.

The Interreg British and French research teams described the same first model in the "grammar schools" in England and in the "lycées d'enseignement général" (general upper secondary schools) leading to the "classes préparatoires". A third school model was developed in the EAZ (Education Action Zones) in the UK (United Kingdom) and in the ZEP, "Zones d'Education Prioritaire" (Priority Education Areas), in France, in socio-economically deprived areas. On both sides the principle of a "positive discrimination" is applied: to give more to those who have less. At the same time, such schools benefited urban policies addressing young people at risk "living outside the school, in their communities, in their districts or towns.

Thus, the school becomes a part of a widened educational community" (Zay, 2005a, p.111).

Even in France, where it is not the main way of working, in Priority Education, more school teams are incited to take into account the students' family and community background. More teachers have educational partnerships with environmental social actors, parents, professionals, sometimes through the parents' working places or projects supported by the local or regional authorities, community associations, elected representatives, etc. But this trend is stronger on British side because the idea of an educational community is better accepted and developed.

A research analysing how school could change in such a new turn could design it as linked with a civil society through its emergent forms defined by Heller (2013, p.2):

> *"The full range of voluntary associations and movements that operate outside the market, the state and primary affiliations, and that specifically orient themselves to shaping the public sphere. This would include social movements, independent unions, advocacy groups, and autonomous non-governmental organizations (NGOs) and community-based organizations."*

Thus,

> *"If services are to be effective, active participation by citizens becomes a key ingredient. Education is 'co-produced' by students and their families. Health is 'co-produced' by patients, their families and their communities"* (p.6).

To Heller (2013, p.2), quoting Sen (1999), at the heart of the concept of civil society is the deliberation introducing modes of mediation among people and organizing collective action. Individual freedom is a basis for seeking a better agreement between all human beings through collective exchanges. To the author the concept of civil society is based on "ideal-type notion that citizens might be able to interact, deliberate and coordinate with each other based on their capacity to reason". Referring to political theorists since Aristotle this process legitimates democratic rule.

In other words, each one learns something from each other and uses his/her capacities to better live with others. They are looking for a win-win. It is why freedom, as conceived in that way, is the basis for equal rights for all. The term freedom here contrasts with it in the neo-liberal paradigm described by Cousins: autonomous individuals use their freedom for their own interests and unequal situations result for each one from being more or less efficient relatively to the others. Those who are more efficient win more. There are winners and losers.

Thus deliberation is both at the heart of civil society and of development conceived as pursuing liberty. Against utilitarian conceptions of development, Sen introduces it by expanding the "capability" of the person "to lead the kind of lives they value and have reason to value" (1999, p.18, in Heller, 2013, p.2). The starting question is: "Can human rights be seen as entitlements to certain basic capabilities?" (Sen, 2005, p.151). They are if we answer that human rights are "rights to certain specific freedoms", and capacities "freedoms of particular kinds" (p.152). Thus to Sen, capability is "the opportunity to achieve valuable combinations of human functioning - what a person is able to do or be" if "she possesses the means or instruments or permissions to pursue what she would like to do" (p.152). Therefore, she needs to be free and to have the right to develop her capability without facing unfair situations like poverty, oppression, insecurity.

As we saw, Sen (2009) explains how the deliberation can only guarantee justice, because everyone has one's own idea of justice, therefore negotiation is necessary to get an appropriate agreement.

But if education aims to prepare the citizens-to-be for such a democratic and inclusive society, it could seem to be using the same principle at school. School would lead them to knowledge by participating in elaborating it through a critical dialogue one with another, between those who have more, the teachers, and those who are learning, like researchers do when they produce a scientific knowledge with their team and other scholars reviewing their results.

Such educational conceptions were developed by researchers and academics in mathematics, experimental and natural sciences, for instance Giordan and its international Laboratory team (Giordan & De Vecchi, 2010).

To Moje (2007, p.1), the central question is: how to resolve the tensions that arise from the intellectual work of teaching content / concepts to people who don't share common intellectual interests while simultaneously enable their full potential- " full lives that might or might not intersect with the content under study". Moje attempts to answer the tensions and dilemmas teachers have to face by analysing current research how "to produce a subject-matter instruction that is not only socially just but also that produces social justice». Her conclusion could illustrate how an inclusive education and an inclusive society need to nurture each other being both supported by the same moral and social justice aims.

> *"The more they (young people) interrogate their practices across all the funds, networks or discourse communities they encounter in and out of school, the more youth can become critical readers and thinkers (...) In this case, teaching with integrity involves developing secondary school subject-matter pedagogy that is socially just in its provision of opportunities to learn how to make sense of and produce the texts of different subject areas and teaches social justice as teachers guide youth in critiquing, challenging and constructing knowledge in those disciplines and in everyday life" (p.37).*

Conclusion

The starting point of the article was an event out of the educational field: the European Union member states adopted a new system of accounts (ESA) including the profits of illegal activities to assess their development. The question was raised: does it make sense to vote such a measure and, at the same time, to claim inclusive education principles, that is to say respecting and giving every one the same right to education? The question included another one: what are the links between education and society, state and other social forces in a globalised world?

To highlight the issues the theoretical sources were research elaborating a conceptual framework to answer contestations against inclusive education promoted by national policies. Through the confluence of social movements, research and international organisations, they point a definition of the concept based on the idea of social justice and "Education for all" versus another based on effectiveness.

Thus, it was decided to analyze the consequences of inclusive education "to accomplish the elimination of exclusion and the positivity of inclusion as a social principle that goes to the heart of the constitution of society."

The methodology follows the authors whose theoretical background inspires mine. To Thomas & Vaughan (2009, p.2), in the last third of the twentieth century, there was a decline in respect for authority, "the culture of 'doctor knows best' (or psychologist or teacher knows best) has diminished substantially". This declining respect has given rise to listening to the users, the parents, the children. It makes sense to compile "a spectrum of voices" and make an issue better understood.

Through this theoretical background and methodology, analysing previous educational research data confirmed the importance of social representations and underlying values for social actors. The DOCA research in ten European countries found the same factor of students' success at school: how much educational staff are motivated and involve themselves to make students successful. The Interreg research can't allow merely opposing state and market or state and civil society. If French policy is supposed to follow the Durkheimian paradigm of solidarity contrasting with the Anglo-Saxon neoliberal view, analysing the French school system highlights that the overwhelming values influencing social actors generate more inequalities in education than in most OECD countries. Under the umbrella of the Republican school the upper social classes capture the public service for their own interests. The public administration and national competitive examinations, the "concours", regulate the game no more and no better than the market in the UK.

These research results were used for extending the issue through other research works, not only about inclusive education and its evolution, but about changing society for making it more inclusive. That leads to the role social movements play both in order to change society and education by opposing another view of society than the ESA example.

But, the associations can favour private interests as well as the public good. Heller (2013, p.5) suggested two keys to distinguish the role played by the associations and the organization of civil society from economic life.

First, are non-profit organisations what they state they are? Are universities "dedicated to the pursuit of knowledge" and "not media just mouthpieces of the state or corporations"? Effort should be directed, on the one hand, towards ensuring both the building of "formal legal barriers and strong professional or normative codes of conduct". In this sense, market power could be considered more a threat to civil society than state power "because as Habermas notes (2001), state power can be democratized; money cannot."

On the other hand,

> *"Creating and promoting an inclusive civil society, and in particular one in which the poor or the socially excluded can self-organize, as such calls for redressing basic inequalities. This in turn translates into a more proactive role for the state and social policy, a role that can be understood largely in terms of providing citizens with basic capabilities."*

So, education remains the key of an inclusive society by giving basic capabilities to citizens-to-be and all along the life.

To Heller (2013, p.6) the way is open to new research about the role of national and international associations in a globalised world could play in rebuilding civil society, thanks to the medium they have, neither power nor money, but communication. It can "shape the exercise of power and in particular can act as a countervailing force to unjust forms of domination" by

- problematization, thus "the women's movement problematized patriarchy", "NGOs and advocacy groups can be seen as part of a civil society infrastructure that routinely problematizes what states fail to deal with";

- influencing or being joined by decisions makers, "It is the civil rights movement that transformed the Democratic Party from the party of Jim Crow to the party of civil rights";

- "holding political actors, corporations, state institutions and other civil society actors to account." The Occupy Wall Street movement illustrates such a case.

Thus the idea of inclusive education and society focuses on the question of human and child rights and the touchstone remains like in the conclusion drawn from the DOCA French report (Zay, 2012a), what Kant (1886, p.41) wrote in 1785 in the scope of the philosophy of Enlightenment: "man and generally any rational being exists as an end in himself, not merely as a means to be arbitrarily used by this or that will."

> *"In the kingdom of ends everything has either value or dignity. Whatever has a value can be replaced by something else which is equivalent; whatever, on the other hand, is above all value, and therefore admits of no equivalent, has a dignity."(pp.49-50).*

Inclusive education and society refer to this ethical aim, the human right to be treated as a human being. For that, it should be a future for a democracy. Indeed so far as a society founded on freedom is continuously moving, always building and rebuilding through conflicts, it needs human values to be recalled again and again, through education of imperfect individual citizens all along life.

Notes

[1] This chapter received the Emerald 2015 Outstanding Author Contribution Award.

[2] Legitimating inclusive education by referring to a link with human rights raises philosophical controversies. In this paper I don't introduce them. I intend to analyze the "strategical" consequence of inclusive education to make society and its school more inclusive.

[3] To be brief, the abbreviation DOCA is used for the international project supported by the European Commission: Lot 3 in tender n° EAC/10/2007: *Strategies for supporting schools and teachers in order to foster social inclusion*, Partner organisation: DOCA Bureaus (Documentatie Onderzoek Coördinatie Advies), The Netherlands. Ten national research teams were gathered together in a consortium to answer the tender. They represented France, Germany, Hungary, Italy, the Netherlands, Poland, Slovenia, Spain, Sweden, United Kingdom (England and Scotland).

[4] http://www.cafepedagogique.net

[5] http://schoolsimprovement.net

[6] http://news.tes.co.uk/

[7] *Poverty and the perception of poverty – how both matter for schooling outcomes,* by Andreas Schleicher, Director, Directorate for Education and Skills, Tuesday, July 22, 2014: http://oecdeducationtoday.blogspot.fr/2014/07/

[8] TALIS: Teaching and Learning in Primary and Upper Secondary Education: www.oecd.org/france/Talis-2013

[9] The British-French Interreg Kent/Nord Pas-de-Calais Project (1999-2001) was planned with the Interreg II Programme supported by the ERDF, the European Regional Development Fund, and extended to 2005-2007 with the Interreg IIIA Programme (2001-2006). Both were led by academics, but included practitioners in a collaborative research. On French side, several of them invested the research in a Ph.D. The aim was to put research at the service of the educational community through a policy of partnerships between researchers and professionals, regional decision-makers and social agents in the local environment. To be brief, the abbreviation Interreg is used for this research.

References

Allan, J. (2003). *Inclusion, participation and democracy: what is the purpose?* Dordrecht: Kluwer.

Allan, J. (2008). *Rethinking inclusion: the philosophers of difference in practice.* Dordrecht: Springer.

Bourdieu, P. (1996). *The state nobility. Elite schools in the field of power.* Translated by Lauretta C. Clough. Foreword by Loic J. D. Wacquant. Stanford: Stanford University Press.

Cousins, C. (1998). Social exclusion in Europe: paradigms of social disadvantage in Germany, Spain, Sweden and the United Kingdom. *Policy & Politics, 26* (2), 127-146.

Derrida, J. (1990). Force of law: The mystical foundation of authority (M. Quaintance, trans.). *Cardozo Law Review, 11,* 919–1070.

Dunn, L. M. (1968). Special education for the mildly retarded - is much of it justifiable ? *Exceptional Children, 35,* 5-24.

Dusseau, J. & Isambert, J.-P. (2003). *Dispositifs-relais et école ouverte.* Rapport de l'IGEN et de l'IGAENR à monsieur le ministre de la jeunesse, de l'éducation nationale et de la recherche, à monsieur le ministre délégué à l'enseignement scolaire, avril 2003. Paris: MEN.

Giordan, A. & De Vecchi, G. (2010). *Aux origines du savoir. La méthode pour apprendre.* Nice, Montréal, Lausanne: Ed. Ovadia, 1st ed., Neuchâtel, 1987.

Goffman, E. (1968). *Asylums: essays on the social situation of mental patients and other inmates.* London : Pelican.

Habermas, J. (2001). *The postnational constellation: political essays.* Cambridge, MA: MIT Press.

Heller, P. (2013). *Challenges and opportunities: civil society in a globalizing world,* Nations Development Programme. New York: UNDP (Human Development Report Office).

Hevey, D. (1992). *The creatures time forgot: photography and disability imagery,* 1-2. London: Routledge.

Kant, I. (1886). *The metaphysic of ethics.* Trad. J.W. Semple. Edinburgh: Rev. Henry Calderwood, 3rd edition, 1st. Ed. Riga: 1785.

King, M. L. (1992). « I have a dream ». In J. M. Washington (Ed.), *Writings and speeches that changed the world.* Foreword by Coretta Scott King (pp.101-106). San Francisco, CA: Harper Collins.

Langouët, G. (2014). *Les inégalités dans l'Union européenne et ailleurs. Et si on osait?* Paris: L'Harmattan.

Lorcerie, F. (1994). Les parents partenaires? *Savoir, 1,* 45-74.

Loreman, T, Forlin, C, Chambers, D, Deppeler, J M & Sharma, U. (2014). Conceptualizing and measuring inclusive education. In C. Forlin & T. Loreman (Eds), *Measuring inclusive education: international perspectives on inclusive education* (pp.3-17). UK: Emerald.

Moje, E. B. (2007). Developing socially just subject-matter instruction: a review of the literature on disciplinary literacy teaching. *Review of Research in Education, 31*, 1-44.

Muskens, G. (2009). *Inclusion and Education in European Countries.* Lepelstraat: DOCA Bureaus 2009: http://members.ziggo.nl/george.muskens/

OECD (2010). *PISA 2009 Results: overcoming social background – equity in learning opportunities and outcomes (Volume II):* http://dx.doi.org/ 10.1787/9789264091504-en

OECD (2013). *PISA 2012 Results: excellence through equity: giving every student the chance to succeed (Volume II),* PISA, OECD Publishing: http://dx.doi.org/10.1787/9789264201132-en

OECD (2014). *Education at a glance: OECD Indicators.France – Country Note,* OECD Publishing: http://www.oecd.org/edu/France-EAG2014-Country-Note.pdf

Rawls, J. (1999). *A theory of justice.* Cambridge (Massachusetts): The Belknap Press of Harvard University Press, 1st ed. 1971.

Rossi, G. (2014). Un PIB sans foi ni loi. *Courrier International.* Paris: UNESCO, 1233, 20-21.

Sen, A. (1999). *Development as freedom.* New York: Knopf.

Sen, A. (2005). Human Rights and Capabilities. *Journal of Human Development, 6*(2), 151-166.

Sen, A. (2009). *The idea of justice.* Cambridge, Massachusetts: The Belknap Press of Harvard University Press.

Thomas, G. & Vaughan, M. (2009). *Inclusive education.* Readings and reflections. Berkshire: Open University Press and New York: Two Pen Plaza, 1st ed.: 2004.

UNDP (2006). *Human development report.* New York: UNDP, 1st ed.: 1990.

UNESCO (1994). *The Salamanca statement and framework for action on special needs education.* Paris: UNESCO/Ministry of Education, Spain.

UNESCO (2005). *Guidelines for inclusion: ensuring access to education for all.* Paris: UNESCO.

UNESCO (2009). *Policy guidelines on inclusion in education.* Paris: UNESCO.

United Nations (1989). *The U.N. Convention on the rights of the child (UNCR).* London: UNICEF.

Van Zanten, A. & Maxwell, C. (2015). Elite education and the state in France: durable ties and new challenges. *British Journal of Sociology of Education, 36* (1), 71-94.

Zay, D. (2005a). Preventing school and social exclusion. A French-British comparative study. *European Educational Research Journal*, 4(2), 109-120.

Zay, D. (2005b). Les paradigmes européens de l'exclusion sociale. In D. Zay (Dir.), *Prévenir l'exclusion scolaire et sociale des jeunes. Une approche franco-britannique* (pp.7-30). Paris: PUF.

Zay, D. (2012a). *L'éducation inclusive. Une réponse à l'échec scolaire?* Préface de Gabriel Langouët. Paris: Ed. L'Harmattan.

Zay, D. (2012b). A secular cooperative school can it promote an inclusive education and society? *Italian Journal of Sociology of Education*, 4(1), 88-112. http://www.ijse.eu

2

Pathways for Inclusion Beyond the School Walls: a Transformative Case of Using Inclusive Education to Enhance Social Inclusion in Spain

Lena De Botton and Ramón Flecha
Universitat de Barcelona, Spain

Rocío García-Carrión
University of Cambridge, UK

Silvia Molina
Universitat Rovira i Virgili, Spain

Abstract

Achieving educational inclusion for all students is still a major challenge worldwide. Efforts to avoid any type of segregation in classrooms and schools have led to a wealth of research on the topic. Although inclusive education and inclusive pedagogy have acknowledged the need to broaden the concept of inclusion, few studies have explored the relationship between educational and social inclusion and its role in guaranteeing every child's right to succeed in education. To study this relationship, this article examines a community-based inclusive approach that demonstrates how an inclusive school model can enhance social inclusion. Building on the results of the large-scale, EU-funded INCLUD-ED project, this school implemented what the project defined as Successful Educational Actions. By describing the improvements these interventions made in diverse contexts, this study demonstrates how inclusive practices in schools led to social inclusion for children and families of a highly socially marginalised school in Spain. The results suggest strategies for implementing inclusion of children and their family members in primary classrooms and reveal their impact on other participants outside of the school. The transferability of these successful educational actions to overcoming educational and social disadvantages in other marginalised areas is discussed.

Introduction

> *I had a period where I was very sick, I was into drugs. I was in a centre for almost 7 months. And then that time, I did not take care of my children. On the contrary, they woke themselves up, dressed themselves and went. Afterwards, I left the centre and I was fine, it was my husband and I.*

This statement was made by Maria, a mother who lives in a marginalised neighbourhood and whose life has long been an example of social exclusion. Her case is not unusual; 24% of all the Europeans (more than 120 million people) are at risk of experiencing poverty or social exclusion (European Commission, 2010a). Maria's story was transformed by her involvement in her children's school. In this school, people dared to dream and created an inclusive environment for children, their families and the community—in Freire's words, they turned difficulties into possibilities (Freire, 1998). The purpose of this paper is to explain how an inclusive educational approach based on community participation in a neighbourhood school improved the educational and social prospects of the school's students and their families' lives.

The relationship between educational and social inclusion has been explored by several educational and social researchers (Avramov, 2002; Bynner & Parsons, 2002). Increased attention has been given to this issue since the global economic crisis began affecting living conditions worldwide (de Greef, Segers & Verte, 2012; Nicaise, 2012). In 2008, more than 80 million people in the EU (16%) lived below the poverty line, including 20 million children (European Commission, 2010a). The economic recession exacerbated this situation. To address this problem, the "EU 2020 Strategy" was implemented to reduce the number of people at risk of poverty to 20 million, reduce the rate of early school dropouts from the current 15% to 10%, and increase the share of the population aged 30-40 that has completed tertiary education (European Commission, 2010b). This strategy represents a challenge for governments, professionals in various social fields and other social agents. EU politicians agree that school systems should be improved to achieve high quality standards and facilitate the social inclusion of vulnerable groups and individuals (Crowley, 2011). Research focused on identifying interventions that can enhance the educational inclusion of all children, closing the achievement gap that affects vulnerable populations, and reducing the risk of poverty can inform public policy and professional practice and achieve the EU 2020 Strategy's goals.

Since the Salamanca Statement (UNESCO, 1994) was issued, inclusive education has played a key role in developing schools and classrooms that offer education for all and creating learning spaces and opportunities that prevent the exclusion of the most vulnerable children. Research on inclusive pedagogy has also emphasised the crucial role of teachers in engaging and facilitating teaching and learning that targets those who experience exclusion (Florian & Linklater, 2010). These initiatives are echoed in the Millennium Development Goals set for 2015 and particularly echo the global aim of achieving quality teaching and learning for all (UNESCO, 2014). However, there is still much to accomplish; there are many pupils from poor socio-economic and minority backgrounds (including migrants, cultural minorities, youth in government custody and people with disabilities) that are heavily affected by early school leaving. In the EU, the average rate of school leaving among migrant pupils (26.4% in 2009) is double that of native pupils (13.1%) (European Commission, 2011). Also, the rate of Roma participation in primary school is substantially lower than the non-Roma average (Crowley, 2011).

Vulnerability is also concentrated in specific geographical areas in most European and American cities. These neighbourhoods, designated "ghettos", contain high concentrations of poverty and other factors that lead to social exclusion. Research has shown that the residents of such areas suffer from segregation, poor urban planning and low incomes (Szczepanski & Slezak-Tazbir, 2007), high rates of unemployment and dependence on social welfare, poor performance and school failure, low quality schools and lack of information about education (Cutler & Glaeser, 1997; Wilson, 2003). They are also at risk to become school dropouts (Crane, 1991) and experience stigmatisation and conflict (Wacquant, 1993). Several of these outcomes are often related to ethnicity (Borjas, 1998). Due to the socio-economic deprivation of these neighbourhoods and their physical segregation within the city, their inhabitants have fewer opportunities for development and are often unable to escape marginalisation and isolation. Although educational inclusion has been used to improve the situation of children living in such conditions (Ebersohn & Eloff, 2006; Kourkoutas & Xavier, 2010), the multidimensionality of the problem indicates that an inclusive approach in classrooms and schools is not enough to solve these communities' problems. More evidence is needed about how this problem can be addressed from a global comprehensive perspective that considers the school and its community context to maximise the ability of inclusive educational initiatives to achieve social inclusion.

Building on the main findings of the large-scale, EU-funded project *INCLUD-ED: Strategies for inclusion and social cohesion in Europe from education* (2006-2011) [1], this study focuses on the implementation of Successful Educational Actions (SEAs) in an inner-city urban school in Spain. INCLUD-ED defines SEAs as educational interventions that have been shown to lead to improvements in educational achievement, behaviour and social cohesion across national and cultural contexts (Flecha & Soler, 2013). These actions have universal components that allow them to be transferred and recreated in different contexts. This analysis focuses on explaining how these

42

actions, implemented in one school, have enhanced social inclusion. More specifically, it explains how SEAs can transform a deprived environment and lead to inclusion for all, even those outside of the school walls. The challenge of implementation and the potential for recreating these actions in other underprivileged neighbourhoods across Europe are discussed.

The role of education in social inclusion

Receiving high-quality education is crucial to guaranteeing the social inclusion of all participants. Moreover, when social inclusion is ensured, greater social cohesion can be achieved. Social cohesion is developed through the social ties created by economic, cultural, political and civil institutions and organisations (Avramov, 2002). The European Union defines social inclusion as "a process which ensures that those at risk of poverty and social exclusion gain the opportunities and resources necessary to participate fully in economic, social and cultural life and to enjoy a standard of living and well-being that is considered normal in the society in which they live" (European Union, 2010, p.3). Educational achievement is considered one of the most important factors in overcoming social exclusion.

It is therefore necessary to implement educational actions that generate equity and overcome social problems, such as segregation, that preclude the best educational results for all, including the most vulnerable (Zimmer, 2003; Brunello & Checchi, 2007, Ladson-Billings, 1994; Orfield, 2001). However, segregation is still a reality in many educational systems and affects highly vulnerable groups of students (Lucas & Berends, 2002, Oakes, 2005). This is apparent in the organisation of "Roma schools", intra-school selection into all-Roma classes, the refusal to enrol Roma students in mainstream schools, and other locally developed informal segregating procedures. In addition, schools with high concentrations of Roma students are generally ill-equipped and understaffed, particularly in the poorest areas. Clearly, students with minority backgrounds in Europe, including Roma and second-generation immigrants, are subject to segregation in their intra- or interschool educational contexts (Szalai, 2011). Segregation lowers performance, incurs disadvantages, and isolates members of ethnic groups.

Moreover, segregated schools tend to be found in urban contexts, reproducing the social inequalities of ghetto life in children's educational environments (Massey & Fisher, 2000; Quillian, 2012; Rist, 2000). Research on social exclusion and poverty have emphasised the multidimensionality of these phenomena. Several studies have attempted to broaden the definition of poverty beyond the idea of economic deprivation (Dewilde, 2004; Sumner & Mallett, 2013). Research has shown that employment, health and social participation are closely related to social exclusion, and these problems should therefore receive particular attention in ghetto neighbourhoods. Precarious labour situations in these high-poverty concentration areas are associated with below-average job vacancy rates and wages for less educated workers (Ihlanfeldt, 1999). Additionally, in ghettos, the strategies usually employed by certain cultural groups to find jobs, such as taking advantage of personal contacts, are less likely to be used (Elliott & Sims, 2001). The effects of unemployment worsen over time. Long-term unemployment has been shown to negatively influence other components of social exclusion, especially economic deprivation and social isolation (Sverko, Galic & Sersic, 2006).

From inclusive classrooms to inclusive societies

Effective interventions for reducing social exclusion and poverty must consider the factors described above and use them to develop action plans. Education research has identified several actions that entail segregation or inclusion in the classroom and described their effects. For example, ability grouping, expressed in measures such as streaming, increases school failure and cultural segregation and damages the cooperative environment in classrooms and schools (Hargreaves, 1967; Rosenbaum, 1976; Wiatrowski, Hansell, Massey & Wilson, 1982; Flores, 2002). Valls & Kyriakides (2013) compared the negative effects of ability grouping (streaming) with the positive effects of actions based on inclusion. Specifically, they clarified the difference between *mixture* and *inclusion* and rectified the confusion in the literature about streaming practices. Their analysis discussed one factor appertaining to streaming, mixture and inclusion: the use of human resources, including teachers and other adults, to support children's learning. Similarly, research about learning processes has widely demonstrated that family and engagement in schools improves children's academic performance and outcomes (Epstein, 1983; Grolnick & Kurowski, 1999; Harvard Family Research Project, 2006/2007; Henderson & Mapp, 2002; Hoover-Dempsey, et al., 2001). Certain types of family and community involvement in schools have been shown to have greater impact on student learning and achievement, including decisive, evaluative and educative participation, which are more effective than informative and consultative participation (Gómez, Munté & Sordé, 2014). *Schools as learning communities* are established only through an inclusive, whole-school intervention that implements these findings to decrease dropout rates and improve school performance and social cohesion (Gatt, Ojala & Soler, 2011). The European Council, among other institutions, has recommended that the Member States develop policies and practices based on the achievements of this inclusive school model (European Council, 2011).

Social exclusion may be overcome more efficiently by addressing the different dimensions of exclusion and by taking into account the agency of diverse social actors. Killean (2003) highlighted the role of equality-oriented non-governmental groups in developing anti-poverty strategies. In a study of schools in ghetto neighbourhoods, Anyon (1995) indicated the importance of coordination among teachers, educators, politicians, religious leaders, activists, etc. to undertake the reforms a neighbourhood needs to escape exclusion.

Wilson (2003) concluded that mobilising cultural minorities and increasing their educational levels were key factors in deghettoisation. Additionally, studies have examined the potential of cooperative school models that promote community development to educate future citizens who support equality (Zay, 2011).

Educational inclusion challenges the historical and social processes that have perpetuated the exclusion of certain groups of students. Critical pedagogy has established a theoretical framework for developing a "pedagogy of possibility" —for creating learning contexts that can be transformed through dialogue, action and reflection (McLaren, 1999; Freire, 1998). Educational inclusion leads to more democratic structures, justice and equality (Kincheloe, 2005). Inclusion can be implemented in classrooms, schools and beyond.

In the case study presented below, educational inclusion disrupted the vicious circle of exclusion perpetuated in a ghetto neighbourhood. Several successful inclusive actions were implemented that helped reverse the situation in this vulnerable context and facilitated the achievement of full inclusion.

Methods

A four-year longitudinal case study was conducted within the framework of the INCLUD-ED project, whose general objective is to study communities involved in learning projects designed to build social cohesion. Each year, the research questions are revised to build on the previous findings and investigate new findings further. This article focuses on the analysis performed in the fourth year of the study, in which the connections between educational inclusion and other types of inclusion were studied. The following research questions were explored:

- How does the implementation of the SEAs create more inclusive classrooms and schools?

- In what ways, if any, does the implementation of SEAs promote inclusion in the community?

The school selected for this case study fulfilled three criteria: a) it served a migrant or minority population with low socio-economic status (SES); b) it was demonstrated to contribute to students' academic success; c) it relied on strong community participation. The school analysed in this article had been implementing successful educational actions for three years and had achieved significant improvements in reducing school absenteeism and increasing pupils' performance between 2007 and 2010 (García, Mircea & Duque, 2010). The qualitative and quantitative data collections for the fourth year of the study were conducted between 2010 and 2011 and are presented in Table I.

Table I. Data collection techniques

Quantitative	Questionnaires	89 Students
		4 Relatives
Qualitative	Communicative Observations	3 Spaces in the school (class, assembly, meetings)
	Open-ended Interviews	4 Representatives from the local administration
		5 Representatives of community organisations
		4 Professionals working on local projects
	Communicative Daily Life Stories	9 Relatives
		7 Students
	Communicative Focus Group	1 Professional working on a local project

The communicative methodology was used (Puigvert, Christou & Holdford, 2012). In addition to describing and understanding the educational and social realities studied, this methodology is designed to create scientific knowledge that can transform these realities. To achieve this transformation, it is assumed that knowledge is created through intersubjective dialogue between researchers and end-users of the research, an assumption based on a belief in the universal capacity for language and action. According to this premise, all collectives can participate actively in the research being conducted about them, including those from vulnerable groups, such as the inhabitants of ghetto neighbourhoods. The intersubjective process of research creates an equitable dialogue between the academy's knowledge and the knowledge of the lifeworld under study. The ultimate goal of the communicative methodology is to identify exclusionary dimensions—those that prevent people or collectives from accessing particular social benefits—and transformative dimensions—those that help individuals overcome exclusion. These dimensions can be identified through critical and egalitarian dialogue between researchers and end-users. Egalitarian dialogue within the research process facilitates a more accurate analysis of the object under study, improves scientific rigour, and ensures the research's social utility as it is permanently validated by the end-users. These features make the communicative methodology the most appropriate for achieving the objectives proposed in this study.

Transforming the school: implementing successful educational actions

The school selected for this case study is located in one of the poorest and most disadvantaged neighbourhoods in Spain. The neighbourhood was created to eliminate the shantytowns inhabited by poor families, who are primarily of Roma origin. After the destruction of the shantytowns, the residents experienced high levels of poverty and earned minimal incomes by performing casual and informal labour, such as selling scrap iron. In 2008, the data showed that more than 35% of the working-age residents were social welfare recipients, 7% were illiterate and 79% had not completed elementary education (Ministerio de Educación, Políticas Sociales y Deporte, 2008). The neighbourhood school was threatened with closure due to conflict between teachers and students, absenteeism, violent behaviour and the community's hopeless disbelief that the education offered in the school could rectify their exclusion and offer better options for the rising generation (Padrós, et al., 2011).

The teachers and the education administration did not feel that these circumstances would change without some decisive action and decided to implement research-based initiatives. They first introduced successful inclusive actions into the classroom by not excluding any students from the classroom and implementing interactive groups. Then, they implemented family education through dialogic literary gatherings, later expanding these actions to other spaces in the school, creating inclusive spaces of decisive participation. These actions had already improved students' school success before the fourth-year data presented here was collected (García, Mircea & Duque, 2010). The objective of this study is to analyse how the actions that led to the transformation of the school also contributed to a neighbourhood transformation.

The school implemented *interactive groups* in its classrooms, a method for grouping students that, according to INCLUD-ED, promotes improved learning success (Valls & Kyriakides, 2013). In the *interactive groups*, students work in small, heterogeneous groups, each of which is mentored by an adult. This type of classroom organisation prevents students from being segregated according to ability and uses the human resources available in the community to support the learning of diverse students. It promotes interaction between students of different levels of ability and from different learning backgrounds and between those with different social, personal and cultural characteristics. Peer learning expands each student's opportunity to learn through a diversity of interactions, ensuring a deeper understanding of the topics taught. This practice increases solidarity among students and makes diversity an advantage. The adults involved in the interactive groups are also diverse, which allows students the opportunity to interact with individuals from a wide variety of backgrounds, including support teachers, volunteers from the community, family members, former students, and other neighbourhood residents. Introducing such diversity into the academic context can also dispel stereotypes about certain social or cultural groups (Tellado & Sava, 2010).

Family education was implemented in the school to allow parents and relatives to determine what, when and how the courses would be held. The results of INCLUD-ED have demonstrated that this strategy leads to academic success. Family education typically entails basic education for families and is closely related to the learning content of the children's classes. Among the more successful activities were the *dialogic literary gatherings* (Flecha, García & Gómez, 2013). In dialogic literary gatherings, adults who have never read a book or are in the initial phases of the literacy process read and discuss classical texts. Family education has an impact not only family members' academic knowledge but also on children's learning (Serrano, Mirceva & Larena, 2010). Parents feel better able to help their children with homework and to contribute to their success. In addition, as children watch their parents learn, they are encouraged to participate more actively in school activities and improve their performance. Parents become role models for their children, and as a result, relationships between parents, teachers and students improve, as does student behaviour. Parents and children can share knowledge and work together at home, thus increasing academic interactions. Consequently, family members develop academic aspirations for their children, which is a key factor in educational progress.

Implementing *family and community participation in decision-making processes* meant opening the school to the community, mothers, fathers and other family members and that teachers would no longer make unilateral decisions about the operation and management of the school and its classrooms. This action can be implemented in several ways, such as through a families' assembly and through mixed committees composed of teachers, students, family members, and other community representatives. In these settings, each member participates through egalitarian dialogue regardless of his or her position within the school. The school under study has advanced towards more democratic participation, which has broadened representation of the school's cultural plurality and allowed the school to utilise more diverse contributions based on participants' cultural intelligence to meet the school's needs (Gómez, Munté and Sordé, 2014). Families' participation leads to more numerous and diverse interactions between children and their families and between families and the school. Children whose parents are involved in the school feel more respect for the school and develop a greater sense of belonging to the school community, which results in lower rates of absenteeism, increased commitment to learning, and, ultimately, improved educational outcomes for children.

These actions made it possible to reverse the situation of the school in a short period of time: the student dropout rate decreased from 30% in 2006-2007 to 10% in 2007-2008. By 2008-2009, dropouts were an infrequent occurrence. The learning results also improved. For example, the students who were in 3rd grade in 2006-2007, when the SEAs began to be implemented, achieved average scores lower than 2 (out of 5) in 6 linguistic competences. One year later, the same students doubled their scores in almost every competence. The implementation of these three SEAs facilitated this progress in the same school in which 6th grade students were once unable to read. Now, students are learning to read at the age of five. The next section will explain how the transformation of the school through the SEAs is impacting not only the children's educational inclusion and academic success but also the adult population of the neighbourhood and other areas of society beyond education.

From the school to the neighbourhood: Transferring SEAs to achieve social inclusion

The success of this school indicated the possibilities, rather than the difficulties, of transforming an inner-city school. The transformation of a ghetto school into a successful school was achieved through the implementation of SEAs, which entailed opening the school to family and community participation. This community-based transformation increased the quantity and diversity of resources available for implementing inclusive educational practices. In turn, the fact that SEAs require the participation of families and the community allowed their effects to be seen both in children's educational improvements and beyond the school context.

Interactive groups

The participation of family members in interactive groups provided a significant source of meaning and transformation for many of them. Before implementing the SEAs, family members were not even allowed inside the school; when the interactive groups were established, they were able to participate in their children's learning. The interactive groups made them feel like agents of change, empowered them and increased their self-esteem. As a result, global improvements have been observed in the lives of the families participating in the school. This was the case for Maria, the mother whose situation of exclusion is described in the opening quotation. Because of her participation in SEAs like the interactive groups, she has undergone a far-reaching personal transformation affecting herself and her children. Maria continued her explanation as follows:

> *And I have not had a relapse thanks to the school, I started coming to the school, to involve myself... for me it is very important, very important! It has changed my life, completely, in all the aspects. Now I am there for my children... For me it has been salvation, to say it here. I think that if I would have not come here I would have fallen again (...) And for me it has been the school, when I started in interactive groups (...) you see how the children learn, how useful you feel, teachers ask your opinion (...) you feel useful, you feel good, you feel valued.*

Importantly, Maria's is not an extreme and isolated case; she is one among many mothers and fathers who have seen their lives change as a result of participating in the school.

Family education

Participating in family education activities improved community employment prospects. Through participation in family education and other school activities, community members increased their own expectations about employment. A member of the community services technical staff described this phenomenon:

> As they [the mothers] are participating in the courses, they have other expectations, different than the previous ones. We need to be realistic because it is difficult now to get a job, but they made a huge change, and they have different expectations. [...] The school must have something to do with that because it is from the moment they have started to participate in it.

Indeed, several employment opportunities have emerged in the neighbourhood as a result of school-related initiatives. For example, in the 2008-2009 school year, the school began offering training to become a school canteen assistant. Women participating in these courses had the opportunity improve their skills, which is especially significant in times of financial crisis. According to the school's data, 85% of the women who participated in the course subsequently found work in the neighbourhood and in the surrounding area. These training courses have created more than 100 jobs in several neighbourhoods. Many parents became officially accredited to assist in social and educational tasks, to be receptionists or to organise educational leisure activities. Additionally, participation in the school has fostered the creation of a network of information and solidarity that reaches even the neighbours that do not participate, as explained by the school's head teacher:

> It is not only for those who are directly involved in the school. The mother of Lucia in the 3rd year, she does not participate in the school but thanks to the

participation in the school of the other people, they have found her a job! Everything is connected.

Several health education activities to improve the students' health were also promoted and implemented through a participative and dialogic approach. Family participation in health literacy increased family members' interest in health and improved their basic skills. Health literacy activities in the school had a positive impact on their decisions regarding certain aspects of their children's health, such as nutrition (Flecha, García & Rudd, 2011). According to the daily life stories of the mothers who participated in these programmes, the skills and knowledge learned through this intervention were transferred to other places beyond the school—into the children's and other community members' homes.

Participation in decision-making

Social participation in the neighbourhood was promoted by offering family and community members opportunities to participate in decision-making processes and management. Dialogic spaces for decision-making, such as the assemblies and mixed committees in the school, enabled families and community members to become involved. The creation of such spaces was essential because it allowed community members, most of whom had never participated in any forum for public decision-making, to participate in the decisions that affected their community. This decision-making model played a key role in incorporating community members' input and demands and promoted engagement in dialogic relationships to reach efficient solutions that met the community's needs.

The school also influenced neighbourhood participation by expanding its volunteering activities and contexts. Participation in decision-making and in other school activities led community members to extend their participation as volunteers beyond the school. A volunteer and sister of one of the students explained how this volunteering improved the neighbourhood:

Besides being here (in the school) as a volunteer, there are people that have also started volunteering in the neighbourhood. They join the workshops for the children in the community centre. There is a reception classroom in the morning, and they play games there, they also go for a walk or a visit, they teach the children how to clean the neighbourhood, and that works as an example!

Even residents who do not have children attending the school feel a desire to participate in it because they perceive its close connection to the neighbourhood and its improvement. Therefore, as the head teacher explained, the school has become a source of mobilisation in the neighbourhood:

There are families who don't have children (...) and they want to participate and they come. They come to have a coffee, they talk about whatever, they talk about the neighbourhood...it's having an impact.

Finally, social participation has been promoted through the creation of the Weekend Centre, which offers educational, cultural, and leisure activities for the whole community, especially the youth, from 5 pm on Friday until 8:30 pm on Sunday. This initiative extends learning time beyond regular school hours through community participation. It has become a viable alternative for children and youth who used to spend their free time wandering the streets. Indirectly, this has also been a successful way to improve the health conditions among the children and youth by preventing them from becoming involved in drug abuse and trafficking, which is a real risk in the neighbourhood. Education also helps prevent certain diseases and has an active role in promoting wellbeing (Triby, 2010).

Transferring successful actions to other disadvantaged areas in Europe

The Successful Educational Actions identified by INCLUD-ED have been shown to result in educational improvements and to transform classrooms and schools in a short period of time. SEAs facilitate the inclusive participation of family and community members and empower students and families to unite and take ownership of their learning experiences. By implementing SEAs, schools as learning communities are preventing early school leaving (European Council, 2011). The case analysed in this paper indicates how the benefits of implementing SEAs can extend beyond the achievement of educational inclusion. SEAs have also transformed and improved the lives of family and community members and their social standards, helping them to reverse the cycle of exclusion in which they were trapped and facilitating social inclusion. This contribution is especially important given that addressing social exclusion and poverty is a priority on the political agenda. The case analysed shows that the social inclusion of an entire community began to improve when SEAs began to be implemented in the school. This may be because SEAs consider the multidimensionality of poverty and social exclusion and developing effective interventions that spread learning processes from the classroom to the school and the community.

The case analysed issues a challenge to initiate and achieve similar transformations in other areas and contexts in which others like Maria are seeking better lives and a better future. INCLUD-ED has shown that SEAs have universal components that have made it possible to develop inclusive education and achieve school success in the many contexts in which they have been implemented; they may therefore be transferable to other schools. However, this process of transferring SEAs across national and cultural contexts should be approached cautiously. Local or national contexts can facilitate or hinder transference, and the challenges and opportunities present in each context should be taken into account. The case presented here is not unique. SEAs are implemented in more than 380 schools across Europe and Latin America. The local and national contexts are taken into account in each case by involving all of the end-users—teachers, children, families, educational administrators, community members— in a dialogue with researchers to recreate these interventions in their own context (Padrós, et al., 2011). *ChiPE*, a project funded by the EU's 7th Framework Programme [2], has led to the implementation of *interactive groups* and *dialogic literary gatherings* in six primary schools in England. By observing the development of these interventions in a wide range of schools, we aim to determine whether these learning environments also have the potential to create a more inclusive epistemic climate (García-Carrión, 2013). Additional empirical knowledge is needed to explain why and how SEAs work in different communities and to what extent they can be effective in other marginalised neighbourhoods in Europe and on other continents. If European schools adopt an empirically sound inclusive model of education, they will not only be able to realise the objective of education for all, but also create pathways for social inclusion and escape from poverty. Success stories from these schools and the families and children whose lives have been transformed by the schools can be used to inform policies and practices whose aim is to not only provide these opportunities for a privileged minority but to guarantee educational and social inclusion for all.

Notes

[1] INCLUD-ED: Strategies for inclusion and social cohesion in Europe from education (FP6, 2006-2011) is the only Social Sciences and Humanities (SSH) research selected by the European Commission for inclusion in the top 10 success stories in research with an added value for society. Retrieved on June 2nd 2014. http://europa.eu/rapid/press-release_MEMO-11-520_en.htm

[2] *ChiPE: Children's personal epistemologies: capitalising on children's and families' knowledge in schools towards effective teaching and learning* (2013-2015). This research is developed at the University of Cambridge. PI: Dr. Rocío García Carrión. Scientist in charge: Dr. Linda Hargreaves. The work leading to this intervention has received funding from the People Programme (Marie Curie Actions) of the European Union's Seventh Framework Programme (FP7/2007-2013) under REA grant agreement n° 332200.

References

Anyon, J. (1995). Inner city school reform: Toward useful theory. *Urban Education, 30*(1), 56-70.

Avramov, D. (2002). *People, demography and social exclusion.* Strasbourg: Council of Europe Press.

Borjas, G. J. (1998). To ghetto or not to ghetto: ethnicity and residential segregation. *Journal of Urban Economics, 44*(2), 228–253.

Brunello, G., & Checchi, D. (2007). Does school tracking affect equality of opportunity? New international evidence. *Economic Policy, 22*(52), 781–861.

Bynner, J., & Parsons, S. (2002). Social exclusion and the transition from school to work: the case of young people not in education, employment, or training (NEET). *Journal of Vocational Behavior, 60*(2), 289-309.

Crane, J. (1991). The epidemic theory of ghettos and neighborhood effects on dropping out and teenage childbearing. *American Journal of Sociology, 96*(5), 1226-1259.

Crowley, D. (2011). *Progress towards the common European objectives in education and training. Indicators and benchmarks. 2010/2011.* Commission staff working document. Brussels: Commission of the European Communities.

Cutler, D. M., & Glaeser, E.L. (1997). Are ghettos good or bad? *Harvard University and National Bureau of Economic Research, 112*(3): 827-872.

de Greef, M., Segers, M., & Verte, D. (2012). Understanding the effects of training programs for vulnerable adults on social inclusion as part of continuing education, *Studies in Continuing Education, 34*(3), 357-380.

Dewilde, C. (2004). The multidimensional measurement of poverty in Belgium and Britain: a categorical approach. *Social Indicators Research, 68*(3), 331-369.

Ebersohn, L., & Eloff, I. (2006). Identifying asset-based trends in sustainable programmes which support vulnerable children. *South African Journal of Education, 26* (3), 457-467.

Elboj, C., & Niemelä, R. (2010). Sub-communities of mutual learners in the classroom: the case of interactive groups. *Journal of Psychodidactics, 15*(2), 177-189.

Elliott, J. R., & Sims, M. (2001). Ghettos and barrios: the impact of neighborhood poverty and race on job matching among Blacks and Latinos. *Social Problems, 48*(3). 341-361.

Epstein, J. (1983). Longitudinal effects of family-school-person interactions on student outcomes. In A. Kerckhoff (Ed.), *Research in sociology of education and socialization*, (pp.101-128). Greenwich: JAI.

European Commission. (2010a). *The European platform against poverty and social exclusion: a European framework for social and territorial cohesion.* SEC (2010) 1564 final. Brussels: European Commission.

European Commission. (2010b). *EUROPE 2020. A strategy for smart, sustainable and inclusive growth.* COM (2010) 2020 final. Brussels: European Commission.

European Council. (2011). *Council Recommendation on policies to reduce early school leaving* (10544/11).

European Union. (2010). *The European social fund and social inclusion* (Belgium: European Union).

Flecha, A., García, R., & Rudd, R. (2011). Using health literacy in school to overcome inequalities. *European Journal of Education, 46*(2), 209–218.

Flecha, R., García, R., & Gómez, A. (2013). Transferencia de las tertulias literarias dialógicas a instituciones penitenciarias. *Revista Educación, 360,* 140-161.

Flecha, R., & Soler. M. (2013). Turning difficulties into possibilities: engaging Roma families and students in school through dialogic learning. *Cambridge Journal of Education, 43*(4), 451-465.

Flores Gonzalez, N. (2002). *school kids/street kids: identity development in latino students.* New York: Teachers College Press.

Florian, L. & Linklater, H. (2010) Preparing teachers for inclusive education: using inclusive pedagogy to enhance teaching and learning for all. *Cambridge Journal of Education, 40*(4), 369-386.

Freire, P. (1998). *Pedagogy of the heart.* New York: Continuum.

García-Carrión, R. (2013). Elementary school children's personal epistemology: contributions for exploring dialogic learning environments. In C. Compton-Lilly (Chair), *Interactive groups: interactive classroom learning environments improving learning for all.* Symposium conducted at the meeting of the American Educational Research Association, Philadelphia, PA.

García, R., Mircea, T., & Duque, E. (2010). Socio-cultural transformation and the promotion of learning. *Journal of Psychodidactics, 15*(2), 207-222.

Gatt, S., Ojala, M., & Soler, M. (2011). Promoting social inclusion counting with everyone: learning communities and INCLUD-ED. *International Studies in Sociology of Education, 21*(1), 33-47.

Gómez, A., Munté, A., & Sordé. T. (2014). Transforming schools through minority males' participation: overcoming cultural stereotypes and preventing violence. *Journal of Interpersonal Violence, 29*(11).

Grolnick, W., & Kurowski, C. (1999). Family processes and the development of children's self-regulation. *Educational Psychologist, 34*(1), 3-14.

Hargreaves, D.H. (1967). *Social relations in a secondary school.* London: Routledge & Kegan Paul.

Harvard Family Research Project. (2006/2007). Family involvement makes a difference, 2. Retrieved from: *http://www.hfrp.org/publications-resources/publications-series/family-involvement-makes-a-difference*

Henderson, A., & Mapp, K.L. (2002). *A new wave of evidence. The impact of school, family, and community on student achievement. Annual synthesis.* Washington: National Centre for Family & Community Connections with Schools. Institute of Education Sciences.

Hoover-Dempsey, K.V., Battiato, A.C., Walker, J.M.T., Reed, R.P., DeJong, J.M., & Jones, K.P. (2001). Parental involvement in homework. *Educational Psychologist, 36*(3), 195–209.

Ihlanfeldt, K.R. (1999). Is the labor market tighter outside the ghetto? *Papers in Regional Science, 78*(4), 341-363.

Killean, D. (2003). Poverty, equalities and social inclusion. *Policy Futures in Education, 1*(4), 626-639.

Kincheloe, J. L. (2005). *Critical pedagogy primer.* New York: Peter Lang.

Kourkoutas, E.E., & Xavier, M.R. (2010). Counseling children at risk in a resilient contextual perspective: a paradigmatic shift of school psychologists' role in inclusive education. *Procedia Social and Behavioral Sciences, 5*, 1210-1219.

Ladson-Billings, G. (1994). *The dreamkeepers: successful teachers of African American children.* San Francisco: Jossey-Bass.

Lucas, S., & Berends, M. (2002). Sociodemographic diversity, correlated achievement, and de facto tracking. *Sociology of Education, 75*(4), 328-348.

Massey, D. S., & Fischer, M. J. (2000). How segregation concentrates poverty. *Ethnic and Racial Studies, 23*, 670-691.

McLaren, P. (1999). A pedagogy of possibility: reflecting upon Paulo Freire's politics of education: in memory of Paulo Freire. *Educational Researcher, 28*(2), 49-56.

Ministerio de Educación, Políticas Sociales y Deporte (2008). *El plan de intervención social de los barrios de la Estrella y la Milagrosa de Albacete obtiene sus primeros resultados* [The plan for social intervention in La Estrella and La Milagrosa neighborhoods in Albacete obtain its first results]. Retrieved from: http://sid.usal.es/mostrarficha.asp? id=13542&fichero=1.1

Nicaise, I. (2012). A smart social inclusion policy for the EU: the role of education and training. *European Journal of Education, 47*(2), 327-342.

Oakes, J. (2005). *Keeping track: how schools structure inequality.* New Haven: Yale University Press.

Orfield, G. (2001). *Schools more separate: consequences of a decade of resegregation.* Cambridge, MA: Harvard Civil Rights Project.

Padrós, M., & García, R., & de Mello, R., & Molina, S. (2011). Contrasting scientific knowledge with knowledge from the lifeworld: the dialogic inclusion contract. *Qualitative Inquiry, 17*(3), 304 – 312.

Puigvert, L., Christou, M. & Holdford, J. (2012). Critical communicative methodology: including vulnerables voices in research through dialogue. *Cambridge Journal of Education, 42*(4), 513-526.

Quillian, L. (2012). Segregation and poverty concentration: the role of three segregations. *American Sociological Review, 77*(3), 354-379.

Rist, R.C. (2000). Student social class and teacher expectations: the self-fulfilling prophecy in ghetto education. *Harvard Educational Review, 70*(3), 266-301.

Rosenbaum, J.E. (1976). *Making inequality: the hidden curriculum of high school tracking.* New York: Wiley.

Serrano, M.A., Mirceva, J., & Larena, R. (2010). Dialogic imagination in literacy development. *Revista de Psicodidáctica, 15*(2), 191-205.

Sumner, A., & Mallett, R. (2013). Capturing multidimensionality: what does a human wellbeing conceptual framework add to the analysis of vulnerability? *Social Indicators Research, 113*(2), 671-690.

Sverko, B., Galic, Z., & Sersic, DM. (2006). Unemployment and social exclusion: a longitudinal study. *Revija Za Socijalnu Politiku, 13*(1), 1-14.

Szczepanski, MS, & Slezak-Tazbir, W. (2007). Between fear and admiration. Social and spatial ghettoes in an old industrial region. *Polish Sociological Review, 159*, 299-320.

Szalai, J. (2011). *Ethnic differences in education and diverging prospects for urban youth in an enlarged Europe. Edumigrom summary findings.* Budapest: Center For Policy Studies-CEU.

Tellado, I., & Sava, S. (2010). The role of non-expert adult guidance in the dialogic construction of knowledge. *Journal of Psychodidactics, 15*(2), 163-176.

Triby, E. (2010). L'éducation à la santé au service du savoir médical : une recherche-intervention auprès de collégiens. *Recherches et Éducation, 3*, 78-98.

UNESCO. (1994). *The Salamanca statement and framework for action on special needs education.* Adopted by the World Conference on Special Needs Education: Access and Quality Salamanca. Spain, 7-10 June 1994.

UNESCO. (2014). *Education for all global monitoring report: teaching and learning: quality for all.* Paris: UNESCO

Valls, R., & Kyriakides, L. (2013). The power of interactive groups: how diversity of adults volunteering in classroom groups can promote inclusion and success for children of vulnerable minority ethnic populations. *Cambridge Journal of Education, 43*(1), 17-33.

Wacquant, LJD. (1993). Urban outcasts - Stigma and division in the Black-American ghetto and the French urban periphery. *International Journal Of Urban And Regional, 17*(3), 366-383.

Wiatrowski, M.D., Hansell, S., Massey, C.R, & Wilson, D.L. (1982). Curriculum tracking and delinquency. *American Sociological Review, 47,* 151–160.

Wilson, W. (2003). Race, class and urban poverty: A rejoinder. *Ethnic and Racial Studies, 26*(6), 1096-1114.

Zay, D. (2011). A cooperative school model to promote intercultural dialogue between citizens-to-be. *Policy Futures in Education, 9*(1), 96-103.

Zimmer, R. (2003). A new twist in the educational tracking debate. *Economics of Education Review, 22*(3), 307.

3

Equity and Quality: Inclusive Education in Australia for Students with Disabilities

Joanne Deppeler
Monash University, Australia

Chris Forlin
Hong Kong Institute of Education, Hong Kong

Dianne Chambers
University of Notre Dame, Western Australia

Tim Loreman
Concordia University, Canada

Umesh Sharma
Monash University, Australia

Abstract

Internationally inclusive education has been variously articulated and interpreted for practice emphasizing both equity and quality in schooling. This article is based on data arising from research commissioned by the Australian Research Alliance for Children and Youth (ARACY) for the Australian Government Department of Education that reviewed inclusive education policies and practices for students with disabilities in Australia. Australia faces a number of challenges if it is to successfully enact all of its stated goals for equity and quality in education. Further, research will need to examine the impact of current neoliberal reform agendas on students with disabilities and investigate professional collaboration initiatives with those in urban and rural contexts to understand how the goals of fairness and inclusion might be achieved.

This paper is based on research commissioned by the Australian Research Alliance for Children and Youth (ARACY) for the Australian Government Department of Education that reviewed inclusive education policies and practices for students with disabilities in Australia. [1] Inclusive education in the Australian government school sector was the identified focus area, and the key research questions for investigation were: How is Australia sitting internationally in relation to the extent students with disability or additional learning needs can access and participate in education on the same basis as students without disability? What are the Australian and international policies (that is the possibilities) for improving learning outcomes for students with disability or additional learning needs? What programs are currently being implemented and what learning needs are they attempting to meet?

To answer these questions, a review of more than 150 individual data sources including: key published papers in peer reviewed journals, publicly available government reports, commentary from internationally accepted authorities and information retrieved from Australian education system websites. We critically discuss some of the findings of the review that arose from the first two research questions and in particular with reference to equity and quality of policies and practices in inclusive education.

Method

We searched for inclusive education policy in ten major education data bases including: A+ Education, Academic Search Premier, EBSCOHOST, Education Research Complete, ERIC, Humanities International, Masterfile Premier, Psychology and Behavioural Sciences, PsychINFO and Summon. The following descriptive terms and keywords were combined using in the searches to maximise the number of potential studies retrieved. *Inclusive education* AND/OR *inclusion*, were combined with *policy* and *disabilities* OR *special education* AND *Australia* OR *Commonwealth of Australia* OR (*names of individual states and territories*) to locate appropriate research. This process was repeated until all possible combinations were exhausted. This search of the literature produced eighty-eight (88) articles and book chapters, which met the following selection criteria:

1. Addressed at least two of the aspects of the research study questions

2. Included specific reference to students with disabilities

3. Source of publication was reputable (e.g. official government website or report, peer-reviewed journal articles)

4. Time range was in the period 2003- 2013 years. In addition, any seminal works prior to this time frame were included. In the case of government policy documents the most recent documentation was included.

The search processes were then repeated using the Google search engine and by going directly to the Australian national and individual state and territories' education department sites and applying the search terms. These searches located an additional thirty-one (31) documents, from both international and national authors (Google) and thirty two (32) documents from government education department sites, which met the selection criteria.

Equity and quality in education

The concept of *inclusive education* has been variously articulated and interpreted for practice (Zay, 2012). Nonetheless, definitions of inclusive education arising from international conventions and legislation share a focus on the right to education and the democratic principle of equity. The challenge for those who are involved in inclusive education has been the linking of equity with quality. The conceptual framework defined in the OECD Report: *No More Failures* (Field, Kuczera & Pont, 2007) and applied in the follow-up study *Equity and Quality in Education* (OECD, 2012) combines equity and quality by arguing that education systems need to be both *fair*, to ensure that personal and social circumstances are not obstacles to educational achievement, and *inclusive*, to ensure that 'all' individuals reach a basic minimum standard of education.

Attempts to translate inclusive education into practice have emphasized equity in regard to access, opportunity, participation and outcomes and the elimination of exclusionary practices that do not serve disadvantaged children and youth. Australia's declared focus in education is consistent with these elements. The first stated goal of 2008 *Melbourne Declaration on Educational Goals for Young Australians* and the companion document *MCEETYA four-year plan 2009 – 2012* is for Australian schooling to promote equity and excellence. *Australian governments must support all young Australians to achieve not only equality of opportunity but also more equitable outcomes* (MCEETYA, 2008, p.16). This goal is made explicit in through the provision of additional resourcing and policies that support high quality teaching, … "essential to student learning and … "critical to creating a high-quality teaching workforce" (AITSL, 2013, p.1). Australian universities must demonstrate that their programs fully address the National teacher standards for accreditation. Despite national standards, there are variations in the curriculum of Australian teacher education programs and some concerns that new graduates may not be sufficiently prepared to respond to the diversity of students in their classrooms (Australian Institute for Teaching & School Leadership, 2013).

Australia's commitment to equity for those with disabilities is articulated through the *Disability Discrimination Act* 1992 and in the establishment of the *Disability Standards for Education 2005* (Commonwealth of Australia, 2006) that clarifies the legal obligations associated with inclusive education. All education providers are required to be aware of and implement the Standards to enable students with disability to receive education equal to that of any other student. In 2008, Australia joined the global effort to promote equal and active participation of all people with disability, ratifying the United Nations *Convention on the Rights of People with Disabilities* (CRPD)

(United Nations, 2006). In relation to education, the convention states that persons with disability should be guaranteed the right to equity of educational access for all students, at all levels, regardless of age, without discrimination and including students with disability.

Unlike other countries with a single educational authority, Australia's implementation of inclusive education policy is impacted by the complexity of the jurisdictional educational systems that exist within its states and territories. While there exists some federal directives, which are linked with funding, each jurisdiction is autonomous in its education policy and education practice. In recent years, there has been considerable debate regarding the need for a national curriculum and assessment program to align the states and territories for enabling greater accountability and a comparative way of measuring student progress (Fenwick, 2011). This responsibility now lies with the Australian Curriculum and Assessment Reporting Authority (ACARA). The development of the *Australian Curriculum* from Foundation to Year 12, in progress, is guided by both the *Melbourne Declaration on Educational Goals for Young Australians* and the *Shape of the Australian Curriculum* (ACARA, 2014). The National Assessment Program (NAP) is provisionally targeted to commence in 2016 with national online assessment. It is proposed that the NAP will support quality teaching and learning; deliver better national and assessment information; and broaden the curriculum coverage of assessments. These various reforms and policy in Australia frame equity in both social and economic terms emphasing "marketised and globally competitive schools" (Savage, 2013, p.186).

Equity in opportunity: provision in Australian states and territories

All jurisdictions in Australia have developed inclusive education policies compliant with the National anti-discrimination legislation and the Disability Standards for education but with different approaches to providing services and different nomenclature used to describe these services (Dempsey, 2011). A review of key policy and provision documents in relation to students with disability from the various government websites as at July 2013 provided a broad overview of placement provisions and in-school supports that are offered by individual jurisdictions (see Table 1). While this paper is limited to reviewing the government sector, the Catholic and Independent sectors also provide education for students with disability. The policies and supports that are offered by these non-government systems, though, vary enormously due to the greater autonomy they experience. In general, supports are similar to those offered in the government sector, although there are more differences at both inter and intra state levels (Cumming & Mawdsley, 2012).

Table 1. Placement Provision for each State/Territory

	Full Inclusion Primary	Full Inclusion Secondary	Full Inclusion Senior Secondary	Partial Inclusion/ Special Unit/ Special class	Partial Inclusion Special Centre	Separate Special School (none or limited Inclusion)
NSW	✓	✓	✓	✓		✓
VIC	✓	✓	✓			✓
ACT	✓	✓	✓	✓	✓	✓
QLD	✓	✓	✓	✓		✓
SA	✓	✓	✓	✓		✓
NT	✓	✓	✓	✓	✓	✓
WA	✓	✓	✓		✓	✓
TAS	✓	✓	✓			✓

Notes:
Full Inclusion – indicates placement full-time in a mainstream classroom setting, with full participation in the curriculum and activities of that classroom (Underwood, 2012). Partial Inclusion – indicates that the student has the option of placement in a special unit or class (or in some instances a number of classes known as a special Centre) that exists within the physical grounds of the mainstream school. Separate Special School – indicates that the students are placed in a setting that is separate to, often physically as well as educationally, the student's local mainstream school. Special schools generally serve students who have moderate to severe disabilities and have specific criteria of entry. Residential School – there are currently no residential settings for students with disability in the State school systems.

Services for students with disability are offered through a variety of settings that include primary, secondary, and senior secondary schools, as well as mainstream schools, special schools, and specialist units in mainstream schools. In some states such as Victoria, there are more than 80 special schools (Principals Association of Special Schools, Victoria, 2009), serving students with a variety of disabilities, including deafness, autism, intellectual disability, and emotional and behavioural difficulties. In other states (e.g. South Australia (SA)) while having fewer special schools (N = 15) have 35 special units, and 85 regular schools which have special classes (DECD-SA, 2013a). There are, nonetheless, broad similarities in the provision of these support services for students with disability across the states and territories. A range of support services such as physiotherapy, speech therapy, occupational therapy and counseling are also provided to students through both government and private providers in all jurisdictions.

While access to separate special schooling options and paraprofessional support is available in all jurisdictions, this may not be equally accessible within and across states and territories. Many authorities are responsible for vast geographic areas that contain a plethora of isolated communities or small regional towns, which have limited access to the range of facilities available in urban areas. For children living in these remote areas choice of schooling may be very restricted, with some only being able to access schooling through 'School of the Air' programs. Access to additional professional support is often on an ad hoc basis for these children and the provision of these services is inconsistent and scant in many regions. Each state and territory has highly structured approaches for identifying students with a disability who require additional support. Complex and varied procedures are developed to support decision making for placements and level of support, with schooling in the regular classroom being considered the first and best option whenever possible. The Department of Education, Tasmania (DoE-TA) *Learners First Strategy 2014–17* states that one of its core values is

'Equity' - the right to challenging and engaging learning opportunities in appropriate settings. A student with a disability is first enrolled at his or her local school initially with consideration for alternative placements being made subsequent to eligibility for registration placement on the Register for Students with Severe Disability (DoE-TA, 2013).

For students who are included in regular schools identification for support is provided through a range of procedures. In Queensland the *Education Adjustment Program* (EAP) utilizes a profile of student needs to determine the extent of additional supports required. Similarly, in Western Australia (WA) the *Schools Plus Framework* (DoE-WA, 2013) adopts six levels of need within each of 11 dimensions and eligibility of students to access special schools in WA is determined in consultation with the principal and the manager of student services. These profiles are similar to the needs-based analyses conducted by other departments of education in other states and territories. In school support varies but is generally provided through additional staffing, multidisciplinary teams, and special programs. In New South Wales (NSW) a report compiled by the Legislative Council (2010) describes a range of learning support to students with disability in mainstream schools that are intended to assist the classroom teacher to adapt and modify curriculum and environments to ensure students with disability can access them appropriately. All jurisdictions further utilize teaching assistants to work alongside teachers to provide in-class support. The role of the assistant is, however, gradually evolving towards a broader class support role rather than the support of an individual child.

A comprehensive range of additional pathways are offered in secondary schools that are closely linked to including students with disability in transitions to post-school options. In NSW the Department of Education and Communities employs support teachers to assist students with a disability and their families to develop a transition plan for post-school options and to connect them with services outside of the school. Within schools, students with a disability, like their peers, may be able to access vocational education training (VET) training programs through partnerships with local Tertiary and Further Education (TAFE) institutions. In Victoria, schools offer pre-apprenticeship programs, school-based apprenticeships and workplace learning. Similarly, in SA well-defined processes delivered through two dedicated transition centres, support secondary students with disability to access transition services focused on "employment training and the development of social personal and community living, skills (DECD-SA, 2013b). Pathways in WA can include various combinations of secondary, vocational, higher and community education, apprenticeship training, informal learning, volunteering, leisure and recreation, workplace experience, and employment (DoE-WA, 2012). In some jurisdictions other government departments provide support for post-school options. For example, the NSW Department of Aging, Disability and Home Care (2013), coordinates a number of post-school option programs for young people with a disability, including transition to work and community participation programs.

Equity in academic outcomes

One of the major challenges in assessing outcomes for students with a disability in Australia is the lack of consistent national and jurisdictional data. In most jurisdictions, students with significant disability have access to alternative or adapted curriculum. The reporting of outcomes from such alternative curricula, however, lack consistency and do not necessarily reflect the 'value' that students may have gained from their schooling. Thus, the outcomes for students with a disability are unknown and are not included in the decision making regarding national and state testing and subsequent planning that takes place around this testing. In regards to assessing outcomes on students' progress through the Australian Curriculum, the Australian Curriculum Assessment and Reporting Authority (ACARA, 2014) suggests that teachers should assess students against achievement standards or against individual goals. Within this framework each state and territory has differing approaches to assessment and reporting for students with a disability. At the time of writing there is no legal requirement for schools to use alternative assessments for students with disabilities, although the Government's 2013 *Review of the Disability Standards for Education 2005* recommended that this be become a focus in future (DEEWR, 2013). This lack of consistency means it is difficult to determine whether appropriate progress is being made by students with varying levels of disability, the outcomes being achieved, or the levels at which they are attained (Cumming & Dickson, 2013). This issue was addressed by the Government's Standing Council on School Education and Early Childhood (SCSEEC) and a new model of Nationally consistent Collection of Data on School Students with Disability was endorsed in a phased approach from 2013 to 2015 (Australian Government SCSEEC, 10 May, 2013). The data will identify "…how many students with a disability study in Australian schools, where they are located, and the level of adjustments provided for them to participate in schooling on the same basis as other students" (Australian Government Department of Education, 2013, Para. 3). The expectation is that the data will support schools to "better understand and implement their core responsibilities under the Disability Discrimination Act 1992 and the Disability Standards for Education" (Commonwealth of Australia, 2006).

In Australia, like many other international contexts, there is increased pressure to demonstrate improvement in academic outcomes through national assessment and accountability regimes despite strong evidence in the US to show they have no effect on student achievement (National Research Council, 2011). Current accountability practices for students with disability appear to be inequitable and to undermine the assessment of significant outcomes potentially achieved during inclusive education. There are indications that students with disability are under-represented in national and state testing and accountability assessments in Australia and that their educational outcomes are, therefore, unknown (Davies, 2012; Dempsey & Davies, 2013; Elliott, Davies & Kettler, 2012). As outlined in the National Protocols for Test Administration, which provide the framework for student participation in National Assessment Program – Literacy and Numeracy (NAPLAN) "… students with significant intellectual disabilities may be exempted from testing. Exempt students are not assessed and are deemed not to have met the national minimum standard" (NAPLAN, 2012, p. vi). Data are provided on the achievement of some student groups (that is, Aboriginal and Torres Strait Islander students and students who have English as a second language), but no data are reported for students with disability (Dempsey & Davies, 2013). The standard of educational accountability for students with a disability appears substantially less than for the regular student body, as many students do not seem to participate in national testing.

Standardised tests such as NAPLAN are founded premises of objectivity and fairness, such that student achievement is completed as a standardised process ensuring that all students complete the assessments under the same conditions. During the *Review of the Disabilities Standards 2005* user and providers from the school sector argued that the practices associated with NAPLAN were exclusionary practices and inconsistent with inclusive education equity practices (DEEWR, 2013, p.46). Cumming and Dickson (2013) analysis showed that implementation processes may not be compatible with the law. Australian students with a disability, *"at best participate with controlled accommodations or are excluded and deemed academic failures"* (p.236). If national accountability testing (for example, NAPLAN) is to remain as a part of the educational landscape, then subsequent measures that allow students with disability to demonstrate that they have gained value as a result of their educational journey should be implemented. In particular, to determine the outcomes for students with significant disability alternative assessment may be required. Compared with national assessment practices in the USA and the UK, Australia's assessment practices are less flexible and do not support equity.

Beyond national assessment, there are strong efforts to reshape curriculum in ways that are important to addressing issues of difference and social equity (Yates, 2013). However, issues of social inequities and schooling are often complex and require more resources than an individual   school can provide to address them. There is increasing interest in developing collaborative approaches to respond to barriers that cross, school, health, social, family, and community systems. There are also moves in many systems to establish greater links and collaboration between special schools and regular schools to provide support for a more inclusive educational system. Arrangements such as school networking (Muijs, West & Ainscow, 2010; West, 2010), university-school partnerships (Deppeler, 2012), and collaboration across systems and professionals (Edwards, et al., (2009), are increasingly suggested as productive ways to build capacity and to avoid "… the fragmentation and duplication created by 'single input services based on categorical funding' when trying to serve individuals and families with multiple and complex needs" (Scott, 2010, p.72). Inclusive education demands the active engagement of multiple perspectives in an ongoing examination and debate about equity, teaching and learning and the quality of schooling. There is little doubt that it is the school leaders, teachers, families, and others directly connected with the issues and challenges of schooling that are best placed to investigate their specific circumstances and to develop innovative solutions for improving and ensuring fairness and quality in their practices (Deppeler, 2014). This process necessarily needs to involve educators in engaging with the general public and with politicians to help them understand how the principles of inclusive education and equity enact with broader educational reform and political changes in the their community.

Equitable funding

Funding linked to categories of disability determines much of the support for students with disability in schools. Although exact figures are not available on what proportion of funds is spent in determining eligibility for special services, evidence from other countries suggests it can range from 20-40% of the total special education budget. Further, a large majority of students who have genuine learning needs do not receive funding (for example, students classified as having borderline intellectual disability or a student with learning difficulty).

Finland is often upheld internationally as a model of progressive and educational excellence, having rated highly on the PISA tests and outranking Australia on global measures of educational outcomes. Prior to 2010 in Finland, support funding was allocated to individual children in what was termed "bounty" funding (Jahnukainen, 2011). This is a similar model to that which has been employed in most education sectors across Australia for a number of years. Subsequently, Finland has adopted a base funding only model which has meant that schools and municipalities no longer receive any extra funding by defining some students as having special educational needs (Kirjavainen, 2010). In contrast, the Review of Funding for Schooling Final Report (2011), known as the 'Gonski' Report (Gonski, et al., 2011) proposed a model of base funding for students, with a loading according to student need, as the preferred method of funding schools to ensure that students with disability and other educational needs will have funding as required, regardless of the educational sector or geographic region. In critically examining this policy attempt to address inequality in schools, Kenway (2013) confirmed that compared with other OECD countries such as Finland, Australia has some way to go in providing high-quality and equitable education and highlighted that "...social advantage and disadvantage and educational success and failure are linked in Australia's school system" (p.21). Further, strong evidence was provided in the Gonski Report to show that socially disadvantaged students, those with disability, and Indigenous students are disproportionately concentrated in government schools and must, therefore, be properly funded. Kenway (2013) argued that a weakness in the Gonski Report was the focus on "… disadvantaged schools rather than on the systemic relationships that also contribute to disadvantage' (p.1). This was echoed by Yates (2013) noting that funding of disadvantaged students can build "… a climate of competitive anxiety that embeds parental concerns about maintaining differential advantage" (p.39). While the model applied in Finland has seen the recent reduction in funding for students with disability to base funding only, there is yet no data on the success of this approach. There is also no evidence to link their model of inclusive education to the success they have achieved internationally in comparative assessments such as PISA. Australia should, therefore, exercise caution in the indiscriminate embracing of any inclusion policies or practices from other countries without due consideration of the application of these to the context of the diverse existing educational systems.

Conclusion

In Australia, national standards for teaching and for curriculum, conceptualise what is important for *all* students to access and the resourcing conditions necessary to support stages of achievement. Meanings and practices associated in Australian education have increasingly conceptualized equity in market terms (Rizvi, 2013; Rizvi & Lingard, 2011; Savage, 2013). Market-oriented notions of fairness and inclusion promote equity based on the assumption that parents irrespective of their socio-economic or other circumstances are able to make choices and obtain a quality education for their children (Savage, Sellar & Gorur, 2013). Special schools are a choice for families in Australia, yet there has been ongoing debate about whether separate special schools are appropriate options for educating students with disability (Florian, 2014). Providing full parental school choice can result in segregating students by ability, socio-economic background and generate greater inequities across education systems. As members of the school sector argued in the DEEWR (2013) Review of Disabilities Standards that:

As schools have been expected to become competitive with each other and to market themselves, we have seen a reluctance to take on children with a whole range of special needs or disabilities, except where that child has very clear resources that accompany them and where there is an expectation that the child will not reduce the school's NAPLAN test scores. The narrowing of the way in which schools are valued and measures of efficiency and accountability have had the consequent impact on discouraging schools from taking on students who are seen to be problematic in a range of ways. (DEEWR, 2013, p.46).

The majority of reform change that has impacted education over the past three decades arises from neoliberal economic theory as opposed to educational theory (Laitsch, 2013). A broader approach is required "… if educators want to "regain control"… and initiate positive change as well as respond to current neoliberal reform proposals" (Laitsch, 2013, p.24).

Australia needs to critically consider national policies in relation to local and regional contexts and jurisdictional practices if it is to enact all of the stated goals for equity and quality. Education policy will need to be firmly embedded and informed by research regarding the specific needs of urban and rural situations, fiscal constraints, support structures, and the capabilities and attitudes of those who are to implement it. Overcoming current inequities in provision and understanding how diversity and disadvantage might be addressed will require collaboration among families, educators and health professionals and engagement with politicians to advocate for change and to build infrastructure to support it. Achieving goals of fairness and inclusion necessitates critical examination of the differential impact of current education policy and associated practices on disadvantaged students and schools. [2]

Acknowledgements

The compilation of these data was originally undertaken for the Australian Department of Education (previously known as the Department of Education, Employment & Workplace Relations), 2013.

Notes

[1] Previously Department of Education, Employment and Workplace Relations (DEEWR).
[2] The government of Australia changed in 2013. At the time of writing, Australia is in a period of rapid policy development that is likely to influence further changes in inclusive education.

References

Australian Curriculum and Assessment Reporting Authority (ACARA) (2014). *Curriculum.* http://www.acara.edu.au/curriculum/curriculum.html

Australian Government Com Law, Disabilities Discrimination Act 1992. http://www.comlaw.gov.au/Series/C2004A04426

Australian Government Standing Council on School Education and Early Childhood (SSCSEEC) *Meeting, Communiqué, 10 May 2013.* http://www.scseec.edu.au/Communiqués-and-Media-Releases.aspx

Australian Government Department of Education (2016). Accessed May 2016 from: http://education.gov.au/nationally-consistent-collection-data-school-students-disability

Australian Institute for Teaching and School leadership (AITSL) (2012). *Australian professional standards for teachers.* http://www.teacherstandards.aitsl.edu.au/Standards/AllStandards.

Australian Institute for Teaching & School Leadership (AITSL) (2013, May). *Initial teacher education: Data report.* Melbourne: Education Services Australia. http://www.aitsl.edu.au/initial-teacher-education/initial-teacher-education.html

Commonwealth of Australia (2006). *Disabilities Standards for Education 2005.* http://education.gov.au/disability-standards-education

Cumming, J. J., & Dickson, M. (2013). Educational accountability tests, social and legal inclusion approaches to discrimination for students with disability: a national case study from Australia. Assessment in Education: Principles. *Policy & Practice, 20* (2), 221-239. http://dx.doi.org/10.1080/0969594X.2012.730499

Cumming, J. J., & Mawdsley, R. (2012). The nationalisation of education in Australia and annexation of private schooling to public goals. *International Journal of Law and Education, 17*(2), 7–31.

Davies, M. (2012). Accessibility to NAPLAN assessments for students with disability: a 'fair go'. *Australasian Journal of Special Education,* 36(1), 62 –78.

Dempsey, I. (2011). Trends in the proportion of students with a disability in Australian schools, 2000– 2009. *Journal of Intellectual & Developmental Disability, 36* (2), 144– 145.

Dempsey, I. & Davies, M. (2013). National test performance of young Australian children with additional educational needs. *Australian Journal of Education, 57* (1) 5–18. DOI: 10.1177/0004944112468700.

Department of Education and Child Development (DECD-SA) (2013a). *Special options and statewide programs for students with disability.* http://www.decd.sa.gov.au/speced/pages/specialneeds/intro/

Department of Education and Child Development (DECD-SA) (2013b). *Transition from school: What is available?* http://www.decd.sa.gov.au/transitioncentres/

Department of Education (DoE-TA) (2013). *Learners First Strategy 2014-2017* https://www.education.tas.gov.au/documentcentre/Documents/DoE-Strategic-Plan-2014-2017.pdf

Department of Education (DoE-WA) (2013). *The Schools Plus Framework* http://det.wa.edu.au/schoolsplus/detcms/navigation/services/the-schools-plusframework/? oid=Category-id-1411453

Department of Education (DoE-WA) (2012). *Transition planning.* http://www.det.wa.edu.au/inclusiveeducation/detcms/navigation/transition-planning/

Department of Education, Employment and Workplace Relations (DEEWR) (2013). *Report on the Review of Disability Standards for Education 2005,* DEEWR.

Deppeler, J. M. (2014). Developing Equitable Practices in Schools: Professional Collaboration in Research. In Jones, P. (Ed.), *Bringing insider perspectives into inclusive teacher learning: Potentials and challenges for educational professionals* (pp.178-188) New York, NY: Routledge.

Deppeler, J. M. (2012). Developing inclusive practices: Innovation through collaboration, in C. Boyle and K. Topping (Eds), *Inclusion in schools: what works* (pp.125-138). McGraw-Hill: Open University Press.

Elliott, S. N., Davies, M., & Kettler, R. J. (2012). Australian students with disability accessing NAPLAN: Lessons from a decade of inclusive assessment in the United States. *International Journal of Disability, Development and Education, 59* (1), 7-19.

Fenwick, L. (2011). Curriculum reform and reproducing inequality in upper-secondary education, *Journal of Curriculum Studies, 43*(6), 697-716.

Field S. Kuczera, M. & B. Pont, B. (2007). *No more failures: ten steps to equity in education.* Paris: OECD.

Florian, L. (Ed.) (2014). *The Sage handbook of special education.* 2nd Ed. Thousand Oaks, CA: Sage Publ.

Gonski, D., Boston, K., Greiner, K., Lawrence, C., Scales, B., & Tannock, P. (2011). *Review of funding for schooling: Final Report.* http://www.deewr.gov.au/Schooling/ReviewofFunding/Documents/R eview-of-Fundingfor- Schooling-Final-Report-Dec-2011.pdf

Edwards, A., Daniels, H., Gallagher, T., Leadbetter, J., & Warmington, P. (2009). *Improving inter-professional collaborations: multi-agency working for children's wellbeing.* London: Routledge.

Jahnukainen, M. (2011). Different strategies, different outcomes? The history and trends of the inclusive and special education in Alberta (Canada) and in Finland. *Scandinavian Journal of educational Research, 55*(5), 489-502. doi:10.1080/00313831.2010.537689.

Kenway, J. (2013). *Challenging inequality in Australian schools: Gonski and beyond. Discourse: Studies in the Cultural Politics of Education.* http://dx.doi.org/10.1080/01596306.2013.770254

Kirjavainen, T. (2010). *Esiselvitysraportti: Erityisopetuksen vaikuttavuus perusopetuksessa* [Report of the preliminary study: The effectiveness of special education in compulsory education]. Helsinki: National Audit Office of Finland.

Laitsch, D. (2013). Smacked by the invisible hand: the wrong debate at the wrong time with the wrong people, *Journal of Curriculum Studies, 45*(1), 16-27. http://dx.doi.org/10.1080/00220272.2012.754948

Legislative Council (2010). *The provision of education to students with a disability or special needs.* https://www.parliament.nsw.gov.au/prod/parlment/ committee.nsf/0/47F51A782AEABBABCA25767A000FABEC

Ministerial Council on Education, Employment, Training and Youth Affairs [MCEETYA] (2008). *Melbourne Declaration on Educational Goals for Young Australians.* Accessed May 2016 from: http://www.curriculum.edu.au/ verve/_resources/National_Declaration_on_the_Educational_Goals_fo r_Young_Australians.pdf

Muijs, D., West, M., & Ainscow, M. (2010). Why network? Theoretical perspectives on networking. *School Effectiveness and School Improvement, 21,* 5–26.http://dx.doi.org/10.1080/09243450903569692

National Research Council (2011). *Incentives and test-based accountability in education*. Washington, DC: The National Academies Press.

NSW Department of Aging, Disability and Home Care (2013). *For school leavers – Post school Programs*. http://www.adhc.nsw.gov.au /individuals/support/learning_new_skills

OECD (2012). *Equity and Quality in Education: Supporting Disadvantaged Students and Schools*, OECD Publishing.

Principals Association of Special Schools, Victoria (2009). *Leading special education in Victoria*. http://www.passvic.org.au/index.shtml

Rizvi, F. (2013). Equity and marketisation: a brief commentary. *Discourse: Studies in the Cultural Politics of Education, 34*(2), 274-278. http://dx.doi.org/10.1080/01596306.2013.770252

Rizvi, F. & Lingard, B. (2011) Social equity and the assemblage of values in Australian higher education. *Cambridge Journal of Education, 41*(1), 5-22. http://dx.doi.org/10.1080/0305764X.2010.549459

Savage, G. C. (2013). Tailored equities in the education market: flexible policies and practices. *Discourse: Studies in the Cultural Politics of Education, 34*(2), 185-201. http://dx.doi.org/10.1080/01596306.2013.770246

Savage, G. C., Sellar, S. & Gorur, R. (2013). Equity and marketisation: emerging policies and practices in Australian education. *Discourse: Studies in the Cultural Politics of Education, 34*(2), 161-169. http://dx.doi.org/10.1080/01596306.2013.770244

Scott, D. (2010). Working within and between organisations. In F. Arney & D. Scott (Eds), *Working with vulnerable families: a partnership approach* (pp.92–115). New York: Cambridge University Press.

United Nations (2006). *Convention on the rights of persons with disability*. http://www.un.org/esa/socdev/enable/rights/convtext

West, M. (2010). School-to-school cooperation as a strategy for improving student outcomes in challenging contexts. *School Effectiveness and School Improvement, 21*, 93-112. http://dx.doi.org/10.1080/09243450903569767

Yates, L. (2013). Revisiting curriculum, the numbers game and the inequality problem. *Journal of Curriculum Studies, 45*(1), 39-51. http://dx.doi.org/10.1080/00220272.2012.754949

Zay, D. (2012). *L'éducation inclusive. Une réponse à l'échec scolaire?* Préface de Gabriel Langouët. Paris: Ed. L'Harmattan.

Inclusion Through Shared Education

4

Inclusion of Students with Hearing Impairments in the Foreign Language Classroom: Insider Stories

Yi-Hung Liao
Wenzao Ursuline University of Languages, Taiwan

Francois Victor Tochon
University of Wisconsin-Madison, USA

Abstract

This study examines how specific experiences of disability (i.e. hearing loss) come into being and how they are articulated within educational practices. It particularly explores issues of social justice and equity regarding the discursive embracement of power relations and situated contextualization of hard-of-hearing students' learning experiences. Foucault's genealogical method was drawn on for revealing the fractured human realities which have formed the hard-of hearing students' learning experiences. The results show of the prevalent governing power reflective of a normative ideological position regarding hard-of-hearing students as deficit learners to be silenced and low achievers to be excluded. This study hopes to play as a starting point to initiate a wide-ranging and provocative dialogue around the issues, concerns, and even fears of the hard of hearing students and educators to provide a more open and holistic environment for the development of effective social justice policies and practices in educational environments.

The focus of this research study is to examine how specific "experiences" of disability (i.e. hearing loss) come into being and how they are articulated within specific culture, milieus (i.e. classrooms), and practices (i.e. education). Inclusive education requires forms of intercultural dialogue, for example with deaf culture (Tochon & Karaman, 2009). We are echoing Scott's (1992) problematizing of the notion of 'experience'. According to Scott, what is important about the rendering of experience is not simply to make visible experiences that were previously invisible, but rather to reveal the ways that experience is not a reliable or self-evident source of knowledge, and that certain discursive regimes allow certain experiences to emerge in history while others get hidden or denied. Scott emphasizes on "the constructed nature of experience" (Scott, 1992, p.25).

Making experiences of disability visible

Looking at the current trend of disability studies and disability rights movement, we can't deny their continuous effort of disclosure and making visible experiences of disability that have previously hidden from history and not been addressed politically. However, while this tendency unquestionably brings to open up alternative modes of being and alternative spaces that most conventional history and politics fails to recognize, it does not necessarily reveal the ways that 'experience' itself is a category of representation that emerges and operates within a particular socio-cultural and historical milieu. As Scott (1992) asserts: "It is not individuals who have experience, but subjects who are constituted through experience. Experience in this definition then becomes not the origin of our explanation…but rather that which we seek to explain, that about which knowledge is produced". (pp.25-26)

Following Scott's conceptualization of experience and considering the nature and importance of this study, narrative research is needed for a deep exploration of such multilayered and textured contours of human disability experiences in education. A strong argument for adopting the narrative inquiry in this study is that life stories provide access to the way individuals constitute self and construct identity (Richardson, 1997). Humans, including people with disabilities, are constantly engaged in the activity of construing meaning. Narrative is the primary means through which humans shape and organize their experience, express their emotions and thoughts, highlight the uniqueness of certain action and event, and ascribe meaning to human lives (Chase, 2005; Clandinin, 2007). Narrative, in short, is a means of coming to know oneself and one's world. Through the act of storying and narrating one's experiences, we are constructing ourselves, and achieving our identities. Therefore, using narrative methods to explore the life stories of the hard of hearing students in this study allows us to investigate the meanings that students ascribed to 'hearing loss' and 'learning' as they constructed their identities. In addition, another characteristic of narrative inquiry is its focus on the dialogical nature of knowledge and its emphasis on the social world as a site where power relations are played out. As such, this allows us to critically examine how the authoritative notions of ableism and hearing embedded around the participants with hearing losses, how the taken-for-granted discourses as learning prevail in education, and how the power relations travel to fabricate the identity construction among hard of hearing students in a site of negotiation and struggle.

Disability identity in the making

Let us have a closer scrutiny to disclose ways of understanding the embodiment of disabled bodies. Central to the studies of disability identity is the paradigmatic shift for understanding the mechanism of power in our society—poststructuralism, for example in Weedon (1997)'s clear introduction, particularly on the issues of language, identity, subjectivity and power. Following Foucault, Weedon (1997) connects subjectivity to discourse, arguing that "subjectivity is produced in a whole range of discursive practices—economic, social, political—the meanings of which are a constant site of struggle over power" (p.21). Using subjectivity to refer to "the conscious and unconscious thoughts and emotions of the individual, her sense of herself and her ways of understanding her relation to the world," Weedon proposes "a subjectivity which is precarious, contradictory and in process, constantly being reconstituted in discourse each time we think or speak" (p.32). Clearly, by Weedon's definition, subjectivity has a more inwardly directed or reflexive essence (her sense of herself) and constantly being reconstructed and reconstituted in discourses. However, it is nonetheless going beyond my purpose here to argue the differences between identity and subjectivity since they are very difficult terms to separate and are often used interchangeably. But to facilitate my discussion on disability identity below, I consider identity as a "cover term" (Ochs, 1993, p.288) and subjectivity as one aspect of identity. After all, given the fact that identity emerges from the interactions of discourses, ideologies and institutional practices (Danaher, Schirato & Webb, 2000; Dreyfus & Rabinow, 1982; Tremain, 2006; Weedon, 1997), the discursive interplay of the different relations of power that normalize and regulate the body is responsible for shaping a disability identity.

Five decades ago, identity or the notions of the self in disabled people have aroused a great deal of interests in medical sociology. Goffman (1963) drew a stark picture of strained relations between disabled and non-disabled people. According to his observations, a major aspect of the disability experience is the ongoing struggles to eschew the potential interpersonal devaluation which has caused the disable individual being classification as less than normal or less than human. If stigma, an attribute that triggers social disgrace, can be minimized or submerged during social interaction through strategies such as using humor, providing competence, or hiding difference, the individual may "pass" as socially acceptable. On the contrary, if stigma cannot be successfully managed, the individual will be expelled to the margins of humanity and oftentimes he or she will internalize the stigmatized, spoiled identity as somehow deserved. In addition, in the analysis of disability as a social role, Scott (1969) theorized that blind people's needs for assistance hold them captive to the dominant philosophies and practices of the blind services system. In the process of qualifying for and receiving services, he maintained, blind people are rewarded for adopting the attitudes and behaviors expected of them by the service professionals, and they are punished for viewing themselves in ways that contradict with the professionals' own views of blind people. Ultimately, they are conditioned to be dependent and compliant, a social role that is systematically acquired under the hegemony of the sighted, as Scott bluntly declared in his concluding chapter, "blind men are not born, they are made" (p.121). Apparently, by focusing handicapping responses of the social environment to human differences, the above two studies have shed light on the issues of impairment and identity into the sociological perspectives.

Although the 1970s was a period of increasingly visible disability rights activism (Davis, 2006; Linton, 1998), many prominent disability scholars began to shift their attention from sociological dimensions to the psychological analysis in terms of impairment-centered and individual-coping framework. Increasingly, researchers (Eisenberg, Griggins, & Duval, 1981; Fine & Asch, 1988) began to attend to the impacts of impairment on the individual's emotional status, the adaptation to impairment-related loss, and the performance of roles, such as worker, student, or family member, rather than on the contribution of society to the creation of disability problems. Noteworthily, empowered by the disability rights and independent living movements, disabled people also have began to accelerate their production and publication of experiential accounts in autobiographies, anthologies, and participatory research reports (Browne, Connors & Stern, 1985; Carillo, Corbett & Lewis, 1982; Duffy, 1981; Zola, 1982).

Until recently, disability studies nonetheless directed the focus more on the subjectivity of disable people, namely the internalization of disability identity. On the basis of his own disability experience and his observations of other, Murphy (1990) concluded that acquiring a disability typically precipitates the loss of familiar social roles and the assignment of a negative identity, such as social burden, object of charity, perpetual dependent, or quasi-human. Moreover, Phillips's (1990) analysis of personal experience narratives from thirty three individuals with physical and sensory impairments led her to conclude that much of her informants' experiences of disability were predicated on the cultural view of disabled persons as "damaged good," a socially assigned identity that they believed was perpetuated by the media and medical and rehabilitation systems. But there are still other studies showing that disabled people are no longer captive receptors of stigmatized identity. In an intensive anthropological study of people with congenital limb deficiencies, Frank (1988) documented their capacity to critique and oppose the negative attributions that bombarded them during the course of development. Instead of longing for normality or covering their stigma to gain acceptance from others who were repelled by their differences, her informants openly presented themselves in public activities and forged empowered identities that integrated disability into their sense of autonomy and wholeness. Later vital studies (Finlay & Lyons, 1998) on the relationship between social categorization and self-concept of people with developmental disabilities also suggest that they, like Frank's informants, can be aware of stigma without inevitably internalizing or even reacting to it. Finlay and Lyons's interviews with developmentally disabled people indicate that although they demonstrate awareness of their labels when asked about them, they generally are not likely to describe themselves spontaneously in terms of disability. Lastly, drawing from a large qualitative-interview based study of the quality of life perceptions of people with intellectual disabilities in Australia, Rapley, Kiernan and Antaki (1998) suggest that the social identities of being intellectual disabled is considered more fluid, dynamic, and heavily dependent upon the social demands of particular interactions. In other words, a person with an intellectual disability can, like any other, avow and disavow such an identity according to the demands of the managing contexts in which they find themselves.

From the above accounts of critical literature on disability identity, the relations between the disabled and non-disabled worlds seem not a small rift of communications, but a deep divide. It encompasses both intellectual and affective components, in that it is based on myth and misconceptions about the experience of disability and conflicting power relations between the disabled and non-disabled people. The gulfs in understanding should in no time be bridged. Recognizing the tension between the disabled and the non-disabled, the present study forges a bridge among the disabled world, the abled world, and the researcher. Shakespeare's (1996) suggests a poststructural perspective for the exploration of disability identity to foreground the objectives and significance of this research study.

Disability identity is about stories, having the space to tell them, and an audience which will listen. It is also about recognizing differences, and isolating the significant attributes and experiences which constitute disability. Some we might choose to change, other to recuperate or celebrate. We may need to develop a nuanced attitude which incorporates ambivalence: towards our bodies, for example. Theory has a part to play in this process. But (metaphorically, if not psychologically), it all starts with having a voice. As Foucault suggests, our task is to speak the truth about ourselves. (Shakespeare, 1996, p.111)

Students with Disabilities in the Foreign Language Classrooms: The significance of coming into world

How do students with disabilities identify themselves in our current inclusive educational settings? Under the impacts of globalization, what are these disabled students' true stories behind the scene? With the trend of foreign/world language education, how do the notions of "language" and "learning" travel to fabricate the construction of the disabled learners' identities? Undoubtedly, time, courage, honesty and ingenuity are of the core necessities to these questions and answers. As Stiker (1999) notes,

> *The one who cracks the code of systems that "make sense" who is least poorly placed to undertake this risky adventure. This is where the gamble occurs, at least in part.... The problem of disability is a bit like the share of pottery discovered during an archaeological dig that justifies important observations on the culture of which it is the vestige.... The moment has then come to try to reconstruct a bit of our culture, on the basis of these fragments. (pp.171-172)*

Recognizing this dangerous game, therefore, it might be appropriate to start with the very organic questions like "what it means to be human?" "What is the definition of leading a human life?" and "what are the ways in which human beings come into the world?" before I start my research journey on investigating hard of hearing students' foreign language learning experiences. In his insightful book titled Beyond Learning: Democratic Education for A Human Future, Biesta (2006) provocatively urges us as educators to treat the question of what it means to be human as "a radically open question, a question that can only be answered by engaging in education rather than as a question that needs to be answered before [I] can engage in education" (p.4-5).

Moreover, the concept of educational learning, according to Biesta, is not just about the "economic transaction" (p.19) of knowledge, skills and values, but is more concerned with the individuality, subjectivity, or personhood of the students, that is of their "coming into the world" (p.27) as unique, singular beings. Following this vein, I came to realize that every individual's coming into the world is neither something that one can do on his/her own nor something being understood as an act or decision from a given situation, given the reason that "in order to come into the world one needs a world, and this world is a world inhabited by others who are not like us" (Biesta, 2006, p.27). As such, everyone is markedly dependent upon him/herself, upon the others, and the contextualized situations in the world. More intriguingly, the very structure of the individual's identity and subjectivity as a singular being can only take place in a "troubling space" (Biesta, 2006, p.53) of social situations. To echo Biesta's assertions, I can argue no more that foreign language classrooms are such a complex "troubling space" that is populated by unique individuals who are so much unlike to one another, in terms of ethnic origins, socioeconomic status, home languages, learning styles and even educational needs. Within this intricate contextualization of foreign language learning, it is all the learners' identities and subjectivities that make everyone into singular and unique beings on the one hand. On the other hand, it is all the human plurality and diversity that are to be appreciated and celebrated to the utmost degree. Accordingly, our role as foreign language educators should not merely be that of a technician or midwife to produce competent or fluent foreign language users, but it is rather our mission as a connoisseur and dreamer to value the difference, uniqueness and particularities of every student's "coming into world" as well as the exposition of human possibilities and justices.

Sketching out the complexity of disability matters

To sum up, in this study we draw on trails of Foucault's genealogical method for tracing the discursive practices which have formed the hard-of-hearing students' present in learning experiences. Foucault has interrogated the boundaries of certain disciplines, and especially the social sciences or, in his terminology, the disciplines of the (hu)man, and he has problematized their methodologies, leaving them open to change. As an alternative to a closed methodology, the genealogical approach can explore the disabled subject in education by locating some of the lost or hidden events and experiences.

The use of genealogy for analysis shows a path out of the theoretical impasses that inevitably appear as a result of a wholesale adoption of general theories and critiques. Genealogy can be used as a critical methodology in the study of disability experiences, particularly deriving from Foucault's groundbreaking historical analyses of punishment, madness and sexuality (1990, 1995, 2003). With the conceptualization of human reality as practices which are to be analyzed from within, many scholars in disability studies have done important work that is genealogical in nature (Baynton, 2006; Campbell, 2001; Davis, 2006). In *Disability / Postmodernity: Embodying Disability Theory*, Corker and Shakespeare (2002) acknowledge that Foucault's work and his genealogical method provide resources for understanding disability:

> *a proliferation of discourses on impairment give rise to the category 'disability'. Though these discourses were originally scientific and medical classificatory devices, they subsequently gained currency in judicial and psychiatric fields of knowledge. 'Disabled people' did not exist before this classification although impairment and impairment-related practices certainly did. Thus social identities are effects of the ways in which knowledge is organized, but his work is also significant for its explication of the links between knowledge and power. (pp.7-8)*

In short, a genealogical approach deals with a vastly different conceptualization trajectory characteristic of revealing the contingent and fractured heritage of human reality and experiences. This approach can also inform teacher education as student teachers are generally unaware of the experiences of these students.

Methodology

By approaching disability and education through the framework of genealogy in this study, we can demonstrate an interdisciplinary methodology that helps understand how disability is enacted within such a complex network of social relations, not just in the past but in the present as well.

Participants

Four hard of hearing students, three females and one male, participated in this study. They were college students at the time of the study. Though entering different institutions, they all were educated in mainstream settings throughout their schooling history. Regarding their daily communication, all participants used voice and residual hearing as their primary mode of communication in despite of the severity of their hearing loss varied from mild, moderate through to severe. None of the participants had other disabling conditions. The diversity of this group of students is shown in the etiology and age of onset of their hearing loss; the age at diagnosis and hearing aid fitting; and the degree of hearing loss. Table 1 summarizes each participant's hearing background.

Table 1: Descriptions of focal participants

P	G	Age 1	Onset of hearing loss	Cause of Hearing loss	Age 2	Age 3	Degree of Hearing Loss
Fay	F	19	Con-genital	Heredity	3	4	Moderate
Eve	F	22	Post-lingual	Medical misconduct	10	10	Moderate to severe
Wendy	F	20	Con-genital	Maternal rubella	1	4	Moderate to severe
Simon	M	19	Post-lingual	Meningitis	6	7	Mild to moderate

Note: P = Participants, G = Gender, Age1 = Age at the time of study, Age2 = Age at diagnosis, Age3 = Age at first hearing aid fitting

Data collection and analysis

Individual, open-ended, semi-structured interviews provided the main form through which data were collected for this study. Prior to the first interview, there was an informal meeting with the participants not only to facilitate the follow-up interviews but also to address ethical issues. The further interviews were also conducted to follow the flow of the participants' narrative comments. All interviews were transcribed and summarized. As discussed above, genealogy conceives human reality as an effect of the interweaving of certain historical and cultural practices, which it sets out to trace and explore with skepticism about the universalistic dogmas of truth, objectivity and positivist reason. Foucault (2003) described genealogy as "the coupling of scholarly erudition and local memories which allows us to constitute a historical knowledge of struggles and to make use of that knowledge in contemporary tactics" (p.8). Genealogy is a way to consider how knowledge or systems of reason change over time as cultural practices (Popkewitz, Pereyra & Franklin, 2001). Central to such analysis, therefore, is to understand how problems of social and individual life become constituted as they do, and change so as to affect the conditions where we live. Put differently, a genealogical approach seeks to trace experiences, processes, and techniques through which truth, knowledge, and belief are produced. It conceives human reality as an effect of the interweaving of certain historical and cultural practices, which it sets out to trace and explore.

Results and discussion

Unmaking individuals with hearing losses as the other

To begin this genealogical research study, it is important to recognize the historical dimensions of human reality in hearing losses, to interrogate the supposed interconnections between reason, knowledge, progress and ethical actions, and to acknowledge the discontinuities and struggling interfaces between various identities within selves, including that of particular hearing/hard of hearing identities, each of which are colored by life experiences and emerge when stimulated by specific contextual situations. The labels of "hearing" or "hard of hearing" do not exist in vacuum as sole entities. From the four participants' narratives of their life experiences with hearing losses, there is one common theme regarding epistemological grounds of "hearing impairments." For them, the term "hearing impairment" has been drawn on modernist cultural territory and social maps of positivist experts or professionals. When being asked to describe their hard of hearing condition in the interviews, all of the participants shared similar stories or situations of multiple oppressions, particularly due to expert professionals' constitutive regimes of ultimate knowledge and power at play.

As early as I was one year old, the doctors brought in the verdict of my abnormalcy... I was just not as normal as others.... I often joked with my mom that these dominating words or advices from the medical professionals were so much like the imperial edict that no one seemed ever to doubt or argue back with them. People just listen and follow them. (Eve)

I was the only one out of the whole family who was hard of hearing, the ONLY ONE, kind of separate and deviant from anybody else... I was the only black sheep with stigmatization because I was hard of hearing. And my memory of childhood is not really a happy one—with lots of doctor visits, hearing tests, and even religious rituals and remedies.... I really don't blame them. But honestly, I feel sorry for them and myself as being such a trouble maker and deviance to this world. (Wendy)

Just because of my abnormalcy, the different hearing conditions, I have to accept all the prosthetics curings which meant to change me into a normal kid, remedy my poor hearing, and bring back to the normal life... Truly, my hearing impairments have made me inferior and blocked me from the normal life. My hard of hearing condition seems to line out a border between the other hearing people and myself. Though this is an invisible borderline, it does prohibit me from crossing and inclusion. (Fay)

All what they said and did was dishearten me and make me question I could act and listen like other normal people, not even to mention going for post-secondary studies. But I have no choice at all in this hearing world because I am just the deviant from the norms in hearing. (Simon)

Obviously, not only the participants but their family members are interpellated by the hearing-dominated views that reproduce deficit perceptions that make them think of hearing losses as something inferior and needed to be remedied and cured. Metaphorically, all four participants, have described themselves, explicitly or implicitly, as having 'impairments,' inhabiting a landscape that is pathologized and marginalized, surrounded by impermeable label borders (Smith, 1999). This end result is the reproduction of reigning ideologies that control the body and mind. As such, the cult of professional expertise has compelled people, with or without impairments, to believe its authoritative voices unquestioningly as a total coherent system of necessary knowledge within a precise territory. The prevalence of discursive politics of power has relentlessly disciplined the so-called impaired bodies, as biological determinations and characteristics to be traced as the objectification and devalued as the other (Foucault, 1995). Consequently, people with 'impairments' are objectified, classified and devalued as "other" in terms of a grand narrative of deviance, lack and tragedy in a dominating hearing world.

New eugenics of ableism and hearing

In what follows, we explore how being a hard of hearing individual is inscribed in time and space. This is literally a space travel, dangerous as all space travels are supposed to be, full of unknown surprises and destinations. The multifarious practices and discourses of the new eugenics of ableism and hearing will be particularly discussed to get an understanding of the intricate identity constructions among people with hearing losses in a way that can inform social justice, equity, and teacher education,

In this able-bodied and hearing dominated world, the eugenics of ableism and hearing has been, consciously or unconsciously, directly or indirectly, prevalent within the very soul of our bodies, lives and society. Ableism is a network of beliefs, practices and process that produce a particular kind of self and body that is projected as flawless, perfect and therefore essential and fully human (Hehir, 2002). To show that hard of hearing peoples' place in society is governed or controlled by the eugenic process of ableism, the participants' narratives of experience are discussed in terms of three discourses—discourses of normalcy, discourses of difference, and the discourses of passing. The focus is on how these discourses are taken up, resisted, rejected, and/or incorporated as the participants construct their identities based on their hearing condition.

Discourses of normalcy

When reviewing the interview narratives, the prominence of discourses of normalcy, both explicitly and implicitly, is unmistakable. In our society, discourses of a prevailing body ideal and perfection exist—the able-bodied, strong, beautiful, healthy, pain-free and productive body (Wendell, 1996). These discourses, including the meanings, representations, images, stories, and statements which construct a particular consensus and understanding of the normal body, permeate the educational structures and practices. Thus, although human bodies exist in remarkably diverse ways, certain bodies are scrutinized and labeled as abnormal or deviant. Negative valuations are ascribed to people with hearing loss by the majority of individuals who take for granted that their own way of being in the world is 'normal'. A consequence of attributing 'normalcy' to hearingness is the construction of those who do not have this ability as abnormal, defective, and impaired:

> *I used to dream about being in a world where being disabled was no big deal, where no one considered it a tragedy. No one thought you were inspiring or felt sorry for you. No one stared at you. I imagined what a relief it would be to be seen every day as perfectly ordinary. (Wendy)*

> *Ever since I lost my hearing, my families and friends, and even any person sitting by me in the bus or subway, walking pass me on the street, have given me the impression that I am not a healthy person… I am abnormal from most people because I don't have a normal hearing. And just because of this hearing deficiency, I will never ever be a normal person and far away from a perfect being. (Fay)*

When I was aware of being the only hearing impaired child in my neighborhood, I felt the sense of embarrassment, shame and inferiority about my hearing loss... And I know no matter how I covered my hearing aids or pretended eased and normally, I am still, and always will not be a normal kid to them. (Simon)

More implicit example of discourses of normalcy at work in the research participants' narratives could be seen in the numerous stories they shared of performing oral and audio identity, in other words, performing normalcy. For example, Fay explicitly stated, "I was what they called an oral success even though I had lost more than 50 percent of hearing in my both ears." Likewise, Simon repeated spoke of his abilities to speak like a hearing person and his exceptional lip-reading skills. He said, "My speech was perfect. I guess people won't believe I am hard of hearing unless I tell them. The way I talk and the voice I sound are just like hearing people, and I am really good at lip-reading too." And Eve highlighted her ability to excel academically in a fully integrated hearing class "on par with the other hearing students."

Discourses of difference

Black bodies, white bodies; male bodies, female bodies; young bodies, old bodies; beautiful bodies, broken bodies; right bodies and wrong bodies; normal bodies and abnormal bodies. Historically, our bodies write our stories in which they have explained our past and framed our futures (Baker, 2002). But it is not our bodies which write the story; rather it is the way in which how we, as a society, construct and perceive our bodies that shapes our history and our future. Put it differently, it is the bodily difference that has determined the social structures and mindsets for centuries by defining certain bodies as the norm, and defining those which fall outside the norm as "the other"; with the degree of "otherness" being defined by the degree of variation from the norm (Wendell, 1996). In doing this, we have created an artificial paradigm of humanness into which some of us fit neatly, and others fit very badly. The discourses of normalcy existed explicitly in many examples from the participants' narrative stories. However, they also existed in other implicit and unnamed ways. Owing to the fact that the very existence of discourses of normalcy presumes the notion of "the other" or "otherness," that is, the opposite of norm, the difference, it was found that a binary relationship intertwined between discourses of normalcy and discourses of difference. The following quotes illustrate the effect of the normalcy/difference binary at work as participants positioned themselves as outsiders, different from the "normal" hearing children.

I didn't really know I had a disability until my first day in the kindergarten. I still remembered vividly that after entering the classroom, I realized that I was the only kid with hearing aid sets. It was the first time I felt ashamed of my hearing impairment because I wasn't like everyone else. I became more depressed and upset when they came over around me fingering "the thing in my ear" and curiously asking about it. (Fay)

Noticing of being different from my other classmates owing to my hearing loss, I felt so excluded and ashamed. All bad ideas and images have been revolving in my mind about myself. At times I felt I was just like the ugly duckling in Andersen's classic children tales in which I was the different one supposed to be persecuted and despised. At time I felt like a black sheep in the class because I could hardly catch up others' sayings and doings. And for most of the times, I felt the hearing difference between me and my friends has built up an invisible wall separating me as an outsider. (Eve)

I was really aware that I was different from the other kids in the schools… No one else in the school had hearing aids. Why did I talk funny? Why did I talk differently than the other kids?… I felt different. I felt like why I was the one to be blamed for my hearing loss? Why did God punish me? Why am I different from everyone else? Why am I alone? The only one? Sadly, this seems to be an unanswered question. (Wendy)

I have hands, legs, eyes, mouth, and ears as others do, a normal person. But when it is my turn to purchase a ticket… I am forced to expose my hidden stigma to the public… All of a sudden, my self-perception as being a normal person is shattered away… I can HEAR their sighing and murmuring. Their expressions of mercy and pity have even made me more sorry for my difference to them. (Simon)

Discourses of passing

The third discourses examined in the participants' narratives were discourses of passing, a theoretical concept used earlier by Goffman (1963). Passing, according to Goffman, refers to the efforts and attempts of the individuals with "discredited stigma" (p.42) or deviant from the norm to act as if the known differences were irrelevant and even nonexistent. Educational settings emerge as a prominent context in the participants' life stories where discourses of passing are at work, influencing how they go about the task of identity construction.

Most of the time, I didn't tell people that I was hearing impaired. I never warned anyone. I just carried on with my life and tried to make it through…At young age, maybe I was kind of over-reacted, but I thought if I told them that I had hearing impairments, they might see me as a morbid and abnormal boy and think of my hearing as a contiguous disease that I would pass it on to them. Or maybe they'd feel awkward and not know how to relate to me. And I really didn't want their pity because I am not hearing well like others. So I never, if possible, told friends that I was hearing impaired. But too bad, they could still find it out though. (Simon)

Sometimes I do felt pathetic and guilty about myself disguising and pretending to others. I know that's not the right thing, but I just couldn't help. Perhaps that's one way of self protection and defense, just like a chameleon, to survive in this hearing world. (Eve)

I was not honest at all about the difficulties I was having. But that was just me. The internal me, the real me, was not like what I told people "I'm fine, I'm okay." I was wearing a mask. Keeping up an appearance and making an illusion that everything was fine. I put on a good front. (Fay)

Lastly, from their narrative stories, all four participants emphasized the added schoolwork that was necessary to do in order to keep up with their hearing peers in class.

I guess one thing about me, as a hearing impaired student in a hearing class, was that I had to work twice as hard. I'd study constantly because I couldn't get all the information as the others did. So it was double the work having to read things all over again and having to make sure that I got it. Or write it again. It was just much more work than you could expect. (Fay)

To let myself more included in the class, I am always working extra hard. It might take one hour for the classmates to finish an assigned homework; however, it could take me one or two days to make it complete. Everything really takes time for me to do. But I do appreciate the understanding from some teachers and selfless help from the classmates. (Eve)

Much more extra work and time on my studies are the only strategy for me to survive in the class. Just because I know I am different from other, I have to work extra hard to make up the gap. (Wendy)

Compared to other students in the class, I have always spent more time and energy on my schoolwork. For example, it seems to be easy for them to memorize a short English poem. But for me, it is really a difficult task to accomplish with hours of looking-up words in the dictionary and brainstorming of memorizing techniques. It does take a lot of extra time and effort, and you won't fully understand the struggles unless you're in the same shoes. (Simon)

Conclusion

For the participants in this study, the variety of hearing levels, the perceived stigma of the hard of hearing labels, their pronounced desire to pass and meld into the hearing world, and the reigning discourses of normalcy and hearing to unmake them as the other, all mitigate the chance of clustering 'hard of hearing' into an easily defined and acceptable neutral identity constellation. Along time, their educational experiences incorporate multilayered levels of interplay between the micro self and the macro cultural, social and historical contexts. With oscillations and disturbances, we see tensions and complexities in the identity construction and commitment among people with hearing losses in their lives and learning experiences.

During the interviews, "silence" is the repetitive episode in their educational learning experiences. The juxtaposition of learning experiences as being silenced by teachers and peers in the classrooms, the silence of an absence of any positive appraisal of their learning outcomes and results, as well as the silent disconnection of curriculum design and support to every individual learning needs. The concept of who one is about is produced in a variety of contextual sites, all of which are structured by relations of power in which the person takes up different subject positions such as student, child, immigrant or disabled person. The normalizing discourses of learning in forms of oral-listening dominated theories or principles have operated to regulate and constrain the identity construction and behaviors of all learners, not to mention the students with hearing losses, and devastatingly perpetuate the regime of ableism. In this study, the prevalent governing power reflective of a normative ideological position regards hard of hearing students as deficit learners to be silenced and low achievers to be excluded. However, it is fairly important to initiate and maintain such a wide-ranging and provocative dialogue around the issues, concerns, and even fears of the hard of hearing students and educators in order to provide a more open and holistic environment for the development of effective social justice policies and practices in learning environments.

In this article, a snapshot was provided, some truths were told, but an urge for reconceptualization of foreign language learning among students with hearing losses is therefore cast. Bringing together a unique collection of personal narratives of hard-of-hearing students' foreign language learning experiences, this study makes visible the presence of disabled beings in the foreign language classrooms and legitimizes their voices, lives, and knowledge to trace and reveal the contingent and fractured human realities which have formed the hard-of-hearing students' disability identity in foreign language learning practices. To answer the pressing research questions, the results of this study indicate the truth of prevalent governing power relations reflective of a hearing epistemological and ableist ideological position regarding hard-of-hearing students as the others to be objectified, deficit learners to be silenced, and lower achiever to be marginalized in the foreign language classrooms. More specifically, the findings of this study have painted a complex picture of hearing disability discourses within the terrain of foreign language practices on the path of globalization by problematizes the existing meanings of disability, debunking the taken-for-granted, and recovering the social, cultural, linguistic, and discursive processes that serve to subordinate hard-of-hearing people by locking them in essentialized subject positions and negatively valued identities while privileging and creating mobile, fluid, valued, multiple identities and subject positions for the other abled and hearing people.

Without questions, nothing would induce more positive change than to grant a voice to the people who know best—the hard-of-hearing students. In this study, the narratives shared by the young participants during the interviews are without fit, dramatic, messy, contested, but affirming. It is only through the prism of their voices and revelation of their life stories could foreign language educators, policy makers, and other players start to interrogate those warps and woofs of difference and sameness constituting the notion(s) of dis/ability in foreign language learning and to further examine the fundamental human and educational developmental issues regarding social justices and human equity. Admittedly, till now, not any prescribed "solutions" to hard of hearing students' foreign language learning have been provided as there is no such an elixir nor miracle to "cure" these issues. However, this study can be seen as a starting point for an empowering practice of making the unknown visible and palpable as well as an ongoing reconceptualization of the great dividing gaps between the presumed truths and lived realities regarding hard-of-hearing students' foreign language learning experiences. The participants herein have been moving us forward to open up entire realms of their lived realities and experiences otherwise left unexpressed or unexplored, to talk openly about it and think critically of a foreign language learning environment being exposed. This study achieved this to a limited degree, and the need for a more extensive and comprehensive investigation and understanding is evident. Indeed, without the timely challenge of the hegemony of foreign language educational establishments, the net effects of disparity between the perceived and lived realities will be the continuation of the hard-of-hearing students' failure to attain the fundamental ideals of social justices, human equality and pursuit of happiness bringing upon the resultant subjugation and underachievement of their potential as foreign language learners and human beings. There is so much work to do in the next journey to listen each voice with the ear of the heart, to ponder the burning issues circulating the discursive constructed notions of "ability & disability," "normal & abnormal," "sameness & otherness," and to further unmask the politics of truth of disability experiences in foreign language education. As such, any so-called "disability," including hearing loss, is no longer a matter of private struggle or public shame but a matter of diversity in learning and living in foreign language learning. This would be so critical and foundational to more effective, sensitive and appropriate foreign language educational policies and practices. Otherwise, the gross marginalization and underachievement of hard-of-hearing students caused by faculty policy and practice is bound to continue.

Acknowledgements

We would like to thank the students who participated in this study.

References

Baker, B. M. (2002). Disorganizing educational tropes: Concepts of dis/ability and curriculum. *Journal of Curriculum Theorizing, 18*(4), 47-80.

Baynton, D. (2006). "A silent exile on this Earth": the metaphorical construction in the nineteenth century. In L. J. Davis (Ed.), *The disability studies reader (pp.33-48)*. New York: Routledge.

Biesta, G. (2006). *Beyond learning: Democratic education for a human future.* Boulder, CO: Paradigm Publishers.

Browne, S. E., Connors, D. & Stern, N. (Eds.) (1985). *With the power of each breath: A disabled women's anthology*. Pittsburgh, PA: Cleis.

Campbell, F. A. (2001). Inciting legal fictions: disability's date with ontology and the ableist body of the law. *Griffith Law Review, 10*, 42-62.

Carillo, A. C., Corbett, K. & Lewis, V. (Eds) (1982). *No more stares.* Berkeley, CA: Disability rights education and defense fund.

Chase, S. E. (2005). Narrative inquiry: Multiple lenses, approaches, voices. In N. K. Denzin & Y. S. Lincoln (Eds), *The Sage handbook of qualitative research* (3rd ed., pp.651-679). Thousand Oaks, CA: Sage Publications.

Clandinin, D. J. (Ed.) (2007). *Handbook of narrative inquiry: Mapping a methodology.* Thousand Oaks, CA: Sage Publications.

Corker, M. & Shakespeare, T. (2002). Mapping the terrain. In M. Corker & T. Shakespeare (Eds), *Disability/Postmodernity: Embodying disability theory* (pp.1-17). London: Continuum.

Danaher, G., Schirato, T. & Webb, J. (2000). *Understanding Foucault.* Thousand Oaks, CA: Sage.

Davis, L. (2006). *The disability studies Reader* (Ed.). (2nd ed.). London: Routledge.

Dreyfus, H. L. & Rabinow, P. (1982). Power and truth. In H. L. Dreyfus & P. Rabinow (Eds), *Michel Foucault: Beyond structuralism and hermeneutics* (pp.184-207). Chicago: University of Chicago Press.

Duffy, Y. (1981). *All things are possible.* Ann Arbor: MI: A. J. Gavin.

Eisenberg, M. G., Griggins, C. & Duval, R. J. (Eds). (1981). *Disabled people as second-class citizens.* New York: Springer.

Fine, M. & Asch, A. (1988). Disability beyond stigma: social interaction, discrimination, and activism. *Journal of Social Issues, 44*(1), 3-21.

Finlay, M. & Lyons, E. (1998). Social identity and people with learning difficulties: Implications for self-advocacy groups. *Disability & Society, 13*(1), 37-51

Foucault, M. (1990). *The history of sexuality*, Vol. 1: *An introduction,* (R. Hurley, Trans.). New York: Vintage Books. (Original work published 1976).

Foucault, M. (1995). *Discipline and punish: the birth of the prison* (A. Sheridan, Trans.). New York: Vintage Books. (Original work published 1975).

Foucault, M. (2003). *"Society must be defended": Lectures at the Collège de France, 1975-76* (M. Bertani & A. Fontana Eds; D. Macey Trans.). New York: Picador.

Frank, G. (1988). Beyond stigma: Visibility and self-empowerment of persons with congenital limb deficiencies. *Journal of Social Issues, 44,* 95-115.

Goffman, E. (1963). *Stigma: notes on the management of spoiled identity.* Englewood Cliff, NJ: Prentice-Hall.

Hehir, T. (2002). Eliminating ableism in education. *Harvard Educational Review, 72*(1), 1-32.

Linton, S. (1998). *Claiming disability: knowledge and identity.* New York: New York University Press.

Murphy, R. F. (1990). *The body silent.* New York: W. W. Norton.

Ochs, E. (1993). Constructing social identity: a language socialization perspective. Research on *Language and Social Interaction, 26*(2), 287-306.

Phillips, M. J. (1990). Damaged goods: oral narratives of the experience of disability in American culture. *Social Science and Medicine, 30*, 849-857.

Popkewitz, T. S., Pereyra, M. A., & Franklin, B. M. (2001). History, the problem of knowledge, and the new cultural history of schooling. In T. S. Popkewitz, B. M. Franklin, & M. A. Pereyra (Eds), *Cultural history and education: Critical essays on knowledge and Schooling* (pp.3-42). New York: Routledge Falmer.

Rapley, M., Kiernan, P. & Antaki, C. (1998). Invisible to themselves or negotiating identity? The interactional management of 'being intellectually disabled'. *Disability & Society, 13*(5), 807-827.

Richardson, L. (1997). *Fields of play: Constructing an academic life.* New Jersey: Rutgers University Press.

Scott, J. W. (1992). Experience. In J. Butler and J. W. Scott (Eds.), *Feminists theorize the political* (pp.22-40). New York: Routledge.

Scott R. (1969). *The making of blind man: a study of adult socialization.* New York: Russell Sage Foundation.

Shakespeare, T. (1996). Rules of engagement: doing disability research. *Disability & Society, 11*(1), 115-119.

Smith, P. (1999). Drawing new maps: a radical cartography of developmental disabilities. *Review of Educational Research, 69*(2), 117-144.

Stiker, H-J. (1999). *A history of disability.* (W. Sayers Trans.). Ann Arbor: University of Michigan Press. (Original work published 1997).

Tochon, F. V., & Karaman, A. C. (2009). Critical reasoning for social justice: Moral encounters with the paradoxes of intercultural education. *Intercultural Education, 20*(2), 135-149.

Tremain, S. (2006). On the government of disability: Foucault, power and the subject of impairment. In L. J. Davis (Ed.), *The disability studies reader* (pp.32-47). London, UK: Continuum.

Weedon, C. (1997). *Feminist practice and poststructuralist theory.* Oxford, UK: Blackwell.

Wendell, S. (1996). *The rejected body: feminist philosophical reflections on disability.* New York: Routledge.

Zola, I. K. (1982). *Missing pieces: a chronicle of living with a disability.* Philadelphia: Temple University Press.

5

Assessment practices of school speech therapists working with cultural minority students: differentiation, standardization and normalization

Corina Borri-Anadon
Université du Québec à Trois-Rivières, Canada

Lorraine Savoie-Zajc
Université du Québec en Outaouais, Canada

Monique Lebrun
Université du Québec à Montréal, Canada

Abstract

This contribution aims to analyze the assessment practices of school speech therapists working with cultural minority students by highlighting the issues they raise with regards to inclusive education. The research conducted underscores first, the obstacles to implementing inclusive differentiated practices and second, the normalization processes at work within these practices. Given the prominence of the psychomedical perspective and the need to take into account the students' ethnocultural and linguistic diversity, how are recognized or reconciled differences and deficiencies?

While inclusive education has attracted far-ranging interest in the world of education and has been the focus of numerous publications in recent years, Bergeron and Saint-Vincent (2011) report on its polysemous nature. Indeed, inclusive education, rooted in the area of special education, is still often conceived as a model for the organization of educational services intended to promote the schooling of special needs students in what is termed the "ordinary" classroom (Conseil supérieur de l'Éducation, 2010). However, "this 'reductionist' conception (…) is not consistent with the humanist and universal objective for transforming educational systems so that it makes them welcoming and accessible to all" (Benoit and Plaisance, 2009, p.8, translation ours). Thus, the aims of inclusive education are clearly larger and more ambitious. According to UNESCO (2009) "the requirement for inclusive schools to educate all children together means that they have to develop ways of teaching that respond to individual *differences* and that therefore benefit all children" (p.9, italics ours). Potvin (2013), on the other hand, defines inclusive education as "a systemic approach that is based on equality, diversity and social justice; it is implemented by practitioners who have assigned themselves the mission of fulfilling the potential of all learners by taking into account their *differentiated* needs (…). [It requires] starting from the needs of the students in order to tailor the services or practices of a system to support the success of all students, particularly the most vulnerable" (pp.10&12, translation and italics ours).

The present article seeks to lay the foundation for a debate on issues concerning the recognition of student "differences" within the practices of school professionals. Although the definition and recognition of these "differences" are the cornerstones of an inclusive approach in education, implementing such an approach poses significant challenges for practitioners. How do school professionals conceive and consider these differences in their practices? And, more fundamentally, are differentiated practices necessarily inclusive? In keeping with our study of this subject and, more specifically, with the assessment practices of school speech therapists working with cultural minority students, we describe, first, the specific context of the Quebec school system and second, the broad lines of the research approach taken. We then present some findings regarding issues related to the implementation of inclusive practices. Finally, these findings are discussed in light of the inclusive approach.

Quebec school system context

School professionals in Quebec currently work with an unprecedented diversity of students. On one hand, we observe that the number of students with handicaps, social maladjustments or learning difficulties (SHSMLD) and the resources allocated to them has steadily risen in the last 30 years despite a smaller school population (MELS, 2010; Tardif & Levasseur, 2010). On the other hand, the importance and diversity of students from immigrant backgrounds in Quebec and Montreal schools is now obvious. Indeed, since the introduction of Bill 101 in 1977 requiring allophone students to attend school in French, the growing cultural diversity has been reflected in schools, notably in the francophone public sector, where such students accounted for 48.13% of the Montreal school population in the 2012-2013 school year (CGTSIM, 2013). Whether these students are different because of the characteristics attributed to them or because of family, socioeconomic or sociocultural realities, they tend to experience "situations (…) that undermine their access to success" (CSE, 2010, p.71, translation ours).

Democratized for now 50 years, the Quebec school system rests on a normative framework that holds all school professionals "responsible for meeting the educational needs of each student in his or her care" (MELS, 2007, p.3). To this end, the *Ministère de l'Éducation* has defined different complementary educational services that call on a variety of non-teaching professionals including speech therapists (MEQ, 2002). According to the *Ordre des orthophonistes et audiologistes du Québec* the speech therapist is a professional of human communication disorders who studies, examines, assesses and treats disorders of the voice, speech, language and the oropharyngeal function using the required assistive technology. Closely linked to the world of education insofar as the tools of their trade – language and communication – are at the heart of learning, school speech therapists have won increasing recognition in recent decades. This is observed, notably, by the profession's involvement in the identification of some handicapped students (MELS, 2007) and by the sharp increase in its practitioners (Tardif & Levasseur, 2010).

In view of the diversity described above and the specific features of the speech therapy profession, our research focused on the professional practices of these practitioners within the context of diversity. More specifically, we explored the assessment process regarding cultural minority students suspected of communication difficulties by school professionals. By doing so, we sought to understand the position taken by speech therapists in terms of their assessment practices vis-à-vis cultural minority students, given the concurrent prominence of the psychomedical approach and the need to take into account students' ethnocultural and linguistic diversity. How, then, are differences and deficiencies recognized or reconciled?

Research approach

To properly define the notion of position as regards speech therapists, we turned to researches in the sociology of education that focused on solving the actor-structure dichotomy. Among these, works falling within a critical and post-modern perspective allowed us to apprehend actor-structure relations more flexibly and with less risk of forming simplistic, deterministic analyses (McLaren, 2007; Torres, 2009). Thus, professional practices, conceived to be at the heart of this relation, recognize the actor's reflexivity and subjectivity while remaining situated (Altet et al., 2013; Fablet, 2001, Tennant, 2006). Since these practices represent not only ways of doing, but also ways of seeing the world and oneself, we used their concrete and ideological dimensions as highlighted by Beillerot (2000). Furthermore, in keeping with the works of Foucault (1975) and, more specifically, his conception of power, we defined the speech therapy assessment process relative to cultural minority students as a "Foucauldian examination", that is, "a power/knowledge area" that "manufactures individuals" (Foucault, 1975, p.200 - translation ours). In addition, the choice of the term "cultural minority students" instead of "students from immigrant backgrounds" or "allophone students" (terms frequently used when referring to ethnocultural and linguistic diversity in schools) is based upon a situational approach to ethnicity that allows us to reject determinisms and focus stakeholders' attention on this otherness (or its external limit) (Gauthier, 2005; Eid, 2007; Juteau, 2000).

Our approach hinges on an interpretive-critical posture (Lincoln and Guba, 2005; Merriam, 2002; 2009) that acknowledges the viewpoint of speech therapists while making it possible to shed light on the power relations that inform their practices. Thus, in-depth individual interviews were conducted with speech therapists (8 cases) working in Montreal primary schools having a large ethnic population. The research also included therapy assessment reports (16 documents) drawn up by the participants. Our analysis employs a threefold approach. The first, *restitution,* which is based on an inductive qualitative methodology and the thematic analysis emerging from the interviews, aims to describe the ideological dimension of the therapists' assessment practices regarding cultural minority students, notably in terms of professional self-definition, conception of these students, practice within a multiethnic context, and the identification of principles of action. The latter were grouped according to the different professional acts that make up the assessment process, to wit: assessment in the student's first language, use of formal tools, informal procedures, case history, establishment of conclusion, and formulation of recommendations. The second approach, *contrast*, describes the concrete aspect of assessment practices based on the decisions and effective actions taken regarding these same professional acts, as consigned in the assessment reports. When these two types of data were compared, five issues emerged that tied in with the five components of assessment. Each comprises two dialectical poles as follows: 1) assessment approach: holistic approach/specialized field; 2) finality of assessment: urgency/renewal; 3) assessment guidelines: criticism/pragmatism; 4) assessment strategies: search for objectivity/clinical intuition; and 5) the cultural minority student, object of assessment: differentiation/standardization. Finally, *criticism* revisits these issues in light of Foucault's concept of "examination" (Foucault, 1975).

For the purposes of this article, we focus specifically on the issue of differentiation/standardization, which examines the implementation of inclusive practices by considering cultural minority students within the assessment process.

Between differentiation and standardization: the difficulty of implementing inclusive practices

The participating speech therapists were quick to recognize several particularities of the reality of cultural minority students and the need to take them into account in their practice, especially during training. The very definition of "cultural minority student" that we obtained is a broad one and includes a plurality of situations such as: recent immigrant, second-generation child, child of mixed parentage, bi- or multilingual child and family's level of knowledge of French or English. The therapists' comments also reveal a fairly alarmist conception of these students' living environment, one characterized by major sociocultural problems impacting their development, notably with respect to language. Thus, the participants offer several principles of action aimed at a more inclusive assessment process. These include assessing the student's skills in the languages he/she is exposed to, using formal tools judiciously, observing the student in different settings, and obtaining relevant information from the parents. These elements show that the ideological dimension of the assessment practices advanced by those who took part in the research leans towards differentiation, which is based on adapting practices to the diverse realities of cultural minority students.

Analysis of the data elicited, however, reveals that the participants rarely implement these principles of action. In fact, their reports reflect a low number of assessments in the mother tongue, few observations in the home, and little recourse to interpreters. In case histories, when particular attention is given to a student's minority status, language is emphasized at the expense of the sociocultural and migration dimensions. Furthermore, we observe few specific adaptations regarding the use of formal tools; exposure to French, recent integration into the school system and the minority context of the first language are largely overlooked when analyzing a student's performance. Thus, in contrast to the ideological dimension, the concrete dimension of assessment practices concerning minority students reveals, rather, a tendency towards standardization of the effective measures and decisions taken.

This discrepancy between the ideological and concrete dimensions of assessment suggests there may be various obstacles to the implementation of inclusive practices. In fact, the participants reported a number of constraints including restricted access to resources - interpreters among them - allowing for assessment in a language other than French, limited time for each student assessment, and the absence of clear professional guidelines. At the institutional level, the organization of educational services for SHSMLD (MELS, 2007) generates practices that, in the words of the participants, prevent them from adopting a genuinely comprehensive approach to assessment. The therapists especially deplore that a student must be identified as handicapped in order to benefit from specialized services, particularly since this identification calls for the use of formal assessment tools and the establishment of a conclusion regarding speech and language pathology that confirms the presence of specific difficulties along with their nature and severity. They maintain that, owing to this situation, the school team tends to pressure them to formulate a conclusion that enables access to specialized services, thereby increasing students' chance to benefit from professional help.

Beyond differentiation or standardization - normalization

We also observe this issue of standardization/differentiation when analyzing the reports conclusions. The establishment of the conclusion is a pivotal moment in the assessment process and reflects the finality of the diagnosis. With respect to cultural minority students in particular, the participants' comments testify to the complexity of this professional act, notably in determining the nature of a student's difficulties.

Understanding differentiation/standardization as regards cultural minority students in light of these considerations leads us to identify two norms referenced by speech therapists during the assessment process. In fact, concurrent with the psychomedical approach that uses a developmental norm for comparing the student's language skills as perceived by speech therapists, there is a second norm, less organic and more social, that makes it possible to gauge the sociocultural particularities attributed to cultural minority students. Recourse to one or both of these norms allows us to distinguish three case scenarios where the assessment process "manufactures individuals" (Foucault, 1975, p.200). In each one, the norm used and the gap between it and the student bring to light "useful differences" (Foucault, 1975, p.216, translation ours), indicating that the student is subjected "to some identities rather than others" (Otero, 2006, p.54, translation ours).

In the first scenario, some assessment reports, which we tend to link to the standardization pole, either omit the sociocultural and linguistic features of minority students in their formulation of the conclusion or attenuate their possible effects. Such is the case, for example, in reports whose conclusion hinges on the presence of atypical developmental manifestations at the expense of other indications specific to students from bi/multilingal contexts, that is, attainment of skills in the first language and protracted acquisition of the second language. Here, the clinical impression of a language impairment appears to overshadow the particularities of cultural minority students, since recourse to the psychomedical norm takes precedence over recourse to the sociocultural norm: the student is medicalized, the speech therapist's conclusion makes the defect "real" by treating it as a physical condition, and sociocultural differences are allowed to disappear since they are, to hark back to Foucault, of little "use."

In the second scenario regarding assessment reports associated with the differentiation pole, the recognition of sociocultural elements renders an understanding of the student's difficulties more complex; it nuances, moderates - even prevents - the establishment of a more specific conclusion. The sociocultural norm is the basis for these reports, which therefore hinders the use of the psychomedical norm. These assessments, during which speech therapists have concluded about language delays or hypothesis of impairments, highlight sociocultural differences deemed too significant to be overlooked in a more specifically clinical approach, as would be the case for language impairment. Here, the distribution around the sociocultural norm recalls the discontinuity perspective where the student's problems at school are explained by cultural misunderstanding between two realities – that of the student and that of the school (Gauthier, 2005). In the participants' opinion, the specific characteristics of cultural minority students (details concerning their immigration experience, multilingual exposure, first language skills or the sociocultural realities affecting their family and community) are conceived here as the constitutive elements of the context of the student's difficulties and can, in certain cases, explain them. In this sense, they represent those "useful differences" for defining a student and justifying, at the same time, the broad and nuanced outcomes of his/her assessment. In contrast to the first case scenario where the psychomedical norm appears to operate to the detriment of the sociocultural norm, the second scenario, which concerns speech and language assessment

117

processes vis-à-vis cultural minority students and is associated with discontinuous sociocultural normalization, appears to delay rather than discount the psychomedical norm. Indeed, contrasting speech therapists discourses and their assessment reports made possible to support the provisional nature of conclusions, leading us to believe that other assessment processes will manage to specify the identity of this "case."

Finally, a third case scenario includes assessment reports where sociocultural elements are viewed as environmental factors that aggravate the student's picture, owing their impact on the severity (not the origin) of the pathology. In these cases, recourse to both norms is observed. The issue here involves assessments where the conclusion corresponds to a speech disorder and where speech pathologies are supposedly "amplified" by certain sociocultural elements perceived to be characteristics of cultural minority students. Thanks to the psychomedical norm, the student is defined by the presence of a defect of organic origin that is inscribed in the body, as Foucault would say. Nevertheless, the sociocultural norm, rather than being discounted, serves to highlight the "amplifying" effect of the cultural specificities attributed to minority students. This is the case, notably, for a student's bi- or multilingualism, which is seen as increasing (but not causing) the difficulties observed. This consideration of the specific features associated by research participants with cultural minority students seems to reflect a deficitary perspective, that is, one that centres on an analysis of the shortcomings attributed to minority students' community of origin (Gauthier, 2005). Thus, recourse to the sociocultural norm in the examination would appear to support the normalization of the minority student. Indeed, the specific sociocultural features put forward in a situation of this kind help justify the medicalization process. As with the use of the psychomedical norm, the "useful differences" clarified by the deficitary perspective resonate in the student's body. They strengthen the organic foundation of the therapeutic conclusion and contribute to normalizing the cultural minority student into a SHSMLD with an aggravated condition.

On one hand, these three case scenarios highlight the importance of the psychomedical approach within the assessment practices analyzed. Although they are based on two norms, the psychomedical norm is, in fact, always present to various degrees, helping to normalize the cultural minority student into a 1) SHSMLD or into a 2) potential SHSMLD or into a 3) SHSMLD with an aggravated condition. In the first scenario, normalization corresponds to foucaldian concept of "normation" (Foucault, 2007), which is based on the use of an hegemonical psychomedical norm determining the frontier between normal and abnormal. In the other two scenarios, the norm is rather created by an interplay of "normalities", corresponding to what Foucault defines as "normalization". It is the case, for example, with the formulation of a temporary conclusion (severe dysphasia hypothesis) that allows schools to grant services to the student without fulfilling all conditions imposed by the MELS. This conclusion enables, by filling the void generated by the established criteria of the SHSMLD identification, to shape a new distribution of cultural minority students with regards to their "useful differences" by the advent of a new "normality". In this sense, according to Foucault (2007)," the operation of normalization consists in establishing an interplay between these different distributions of normality and [in] acting to bring the most unfavorable in line with the more favorable. [...] These distributions will serve as the norm" (p.69).

On the other hand, these scenarios allow us to view differentiation/standardization differently. Although they appear at first glance to be in opposition, the two poles are actually in a dialectical relationship, where differentiation and standardization constitute the two dimensions of a same reality, normalization. Diversity is reduced to these "useful differences", those the school may take into account, and their consideration both differentiates and standardizes during a process in which the cultural minority student, normalized, is assigned a new identity, "a second specific, positive and analytical 'reality'" (Otero, 2006, p.11, translation ours) for purposes of social regulation.

Conclusion

Our approach first underscored the obstacles encountered by speech therapists in the process of implementing practices termed inclusive. Consistent with an inclusive education aimed at promoting the dignity of the student, it becomes necessary to remove the impediments to the implementation of comprehensive assessment practices, which are characterized by their credibility and effectiveness in terms of the realities and experiences of cultural minority students (Zay, 2012). Nevertheless, the recognition of the assessment process as a Foucauldian examination changed the debate on therapists and their practices to one on the discourse of truth underlying these practices and allowing the regulation of "behaviours that "pose a problem" (Otero, 2006, p.51, translation ours). In consequence, subsequent analyses will make possible to move beyond these first considerations and will shed light on the importance of the psychomedical approach within the assessment processes regarding cultural minority students and on how this approach fits into the normalization process. To promote the student's dignity (Zay, 2012), inclusive education cannot, in our opinion, dispense with the overriding importance of this approach because "the inclusive school is the one that goes beyond normalization" (Rousseau & Prud'homme, 2010, p.10, translation ours). In this respect, "inclusion does not imply departing from the school and social norm, it implies deconstructing them" (Benoit & Plaisance, 2009, p.8, translation ours).

Notes

[1] There is agreement in both Quebec and Canada on qualifying "allophones" as individuals whose mother tongue is not French, English or a North American Indian language. The mother tongue is defined as the "first language learned at home in childhood and still understood by the individual on May 10, 2011" (Statistics Canada 2013, unpaged document).

[2] Indeed, the effects of Bill 101 were quick to be seen. Between 1980 and 1990, the percentage of allophones directed to the French school network passed from 39% to 75% (Conseil de la langue française [CLF], 1992, cited in Bourhis, 1993). This percentage even exceeded 80% between 1995 and 1998 (MEQ, 1999).

[3] Consistent with our theoretical choices, we did not offer participants a prior definition of "cultural minority students".

[4] The term "amplified" is used by the speech therapists themselves in several reports.

References

Altet, M., Desjardins, J., Étienne, R., Paquay, L., & Perrenoud, P. (Eds) (2013). *Former des enseignants réflexifs*. Paris: L'Harmattan.

Beillerot, J. (2000). L'analyse des pratiques professionnelles: pourquoi cette expression. In C. Blanchard-Laville & Fablet, D. (Eds), *Analyser les pratiques professionnelles* (pp.21-28). Paris: L'Harmattan.

Benoit, H., & Plaisance, E. (2009). L'éducation inclusive en France et dans le monde: présentation. *La nouvelle revue de l'adaptation et de la scolarisation, Hors série* (5), 3-8.

Bergeron, G., & Saint-Vincent, L. (2011). L'intégration scolaire au Québec: regard exploratoire sur les défis de la formation à l'enseignement au primaire et au préscolaire. *Éducation et francophonie, 39*, 272-295.

Bourhis, R.Y. (1994). Ethnic and language attitudes in Quebec. In J. W. Berry & J. A. Laponce (Eds), *Ethnicity and culture in Canada: the research landscape* (pp.322-360). Toronto: University of Toronto Press.

Conseil de gestion de la taxe scolaire de l'île de Montréal (CGTSIM) (2013). *Portrait socioculturel des élèves inscrits dans les écoles publiques de l'île de Montréal, inscriptions au 7 novembre 2012*. Montréal: CGTSIM.

Conseil supérieur de l'éducation (CSÉ) (2010). *Conjuguer équité et performance en éducation, un défi de société*. Québec, Gouvernement du Québec.

Dionne, C., & Rousseau, N. (2006). *Transformation des pratiques éducatives: La recherche sur l'inclusion scolaire*. Québec: Presses de l'Université du Québec

Eid, P. (2007). *Being Arab: ethnic and religious identity building among second generation youth in Montreal.* Montreal, Kinston: McGill-Queen's University Press.

Fablet, D. (2001). Les apports des pratiques d'orientation psychosociologique. In C. Blanchard-Laville & D. Fablet (Eds), *Sources théoriques et techniques de l'analyse des pratiques professionnelles* (pp.151-169). Paris: L'Harmattan.

Foucault, M. (1975). *Surveiller et punir: naissance de la prison.* Paris: Gallimard.

Foucault, M. (2007). *Security, territory, population.* New York: Palgrave Macmillan.

Frandji, D., Pincemin, J.-M., Demeuse, M., Greger, D., & Rochex, J.-Y. (Eds.). *Comparaison des politiques d'éducation prioritaire en Europe. Rapport scientifique, vol. 2: éléments d'une analyse transversale: formes de ciblage, action, évaluation.* Lyon: Institut National de Recherche Pédagogique.

Gauthier, R. (2005). *Le rapport à l'institution scolaire chez de jeunes amérindiens en fin de formation secondaire: contribution à la compréhension du cheminement scolaire chez les Autochtones.* Thèse de doctorat inédite, Sciences de l'Éducation, Université du Québec à Chicoutimi.

Juteau, D. (2000). *L'ethnicité et ses frontières.* Montréal: Presses de l'Université de Montréal.

Lincoln, Y. S., & Guba, E. G. (2005). Paradigmatic controversies, contradictions, and emerging confluences. In N. K. Denzin & Y. S. Lincoln (Eds), *Handbook of qualitative research* (pp.97-127). Thousand Oaks: Sage.

McLaren, P. (2007). *Life in schools: an introduction to critical pedagogy in the foundations of education.* New York: Allyn and Bacon.

Merriam, S. B. (2009). *Qualitative research: a guide to design implementation.* San Francisco: Jossey-Bass Publishers.

Merriam, S. B. (2002). *Qualitative research in practice.* San Franscisco: Jossey-Bass.

Ministère de l'Éducation (MEQ), Gouvernement du Québec (2002). *Les services éducatifs complémentaires: essentiels à la réussite/Complementary educational services: essential to success.* Québec: Direction de la formation générale des jeunes.

Ministère de l'Éducation (MEQ), Gouvernement du Québec (1999). *La situation linguistique dans le secteur de l'éducation en 1997-1998/The linguistic situation in the education sector, 1997-98.* Québec: Direction des études statistiques et des études quantitatives.

Ministère de l'Éducation, du Loisir et du Sport (MELS), Gouvernement du Québec (2010). *Rencontre des partenaires en éducation. Document d'appui à la réflexion. Rencontre sur l'intégration des élèves handicapés ou en difficulté, 25 octobre*

2010. Retrieved from: http://www.mels.gouv.qc.ca/sections/ publications/publications/EPEPS/Formation_jeunes/Adaptation_scola ire/RencontrePartEduc_DocAppuiReflexion_RencIntegrationElevesHa ndDiff.pdf.

Ministère de l'Éducation, du Loisir et du Sport (MELS), Gouvernement du Québec (2007). *L'organisation des services éducatifs aux élèves à risque et aux élèves handicapés ou en difficulté d'adaptation ou d'apprentissage (EHDAA)/Organization of educational services for at-risk students and students with handicaps, social maladjustments or learning difficulties (SHSMLD).* Québec: Direction de l'adaptation scolaire.

Ordre des Orthophonistes et Audiologistes du Québec (OOAQ) (1998). *Audiologiste et orthophoniste deux professionnels de la communication.* Retrieved from http://www.ooaq.qc.ca/Info/pgRoleOA.html.

Otero, M. (2006). La sociologie de Michel Foucault: une critique de la raison impure. *Sociologie et sociétés, 38*(2), 49-72.

Potvin, M. (2013). L'éducation inclusive et antidiscriminatoire: fondements et perspectives. In M. Mc Andrew, M. Potvin & C. Borri-Anadon (Eds), *Le développement d'institutions inclusives en contexte de diversité* (pp.9-26). Québec: Presses de l'Université du Québec.

Rousseau, N. & Prud'homme, L. (2010). C'est mon école à moi aussi... Caractéristiques essentielles de l'école inclusive. In N. Rousseau (Ed.), *La pédagogie de l'inclusion scolaire: pistes d'action pour apprendre tous ensemble* (pp.7-46). Québec: Presses de l'Université du Québec.

Statistics Canada (2013). *National household survey dictionary 2011.* Catalogue number 99-000-XWE in Statistics Canada database.

Tardif, M., & Levasseur, L. (2010). *La division du travail éducatif: une perspective nord-américaine.* Paris: Presses Universitaires de France.

Tennant. M. (2006). *Psychology and adult learning.* New York: Routledge.

Torres, C. A. (2009). *Education and neoliberal globalization.* New York: Routledge.

UNESCO (2009). *Policy guidelines on inclusion in education.* Paris, France: United Nations Educational, Scientific and Cultural Organization.

Zay, D. (2012). *L'éducation inclusive. Une réponse à l'échec scolaire?* Préface de Gabriel Langouët. Paris: L'Harmattan.

The Children in Specialised Classes in Primary School: Between Integration and Inclusion

Claire de Saint Martin
Université de Cergy Pontoise, France

Abstract

In French primary schools, children with disabilities can be admitted collectively to a specialised class, called "Class for School Inclusion" (CLIS). CLIS 1 are designed specifically for children with cognitive disabilities. In the CLIS, they receive personalised teaching, and participate in their respective regular class for specific lessons. The extent of inclusion in their regular classes is specific to each child. This paper reports one doctoral research seeking to understand the place of these children in the school, as they experience it, from what they say. The establishment of a socio-clinical device has allowed the construction of a collective reflection with children from three different CLIS. These reflections, combined with participant observations, allow us to see the issues of school inclusion for the children in these three schools.

In France, the 2005 law "For the equality of rights and opportunities, participation and citizenship of handicapped people" established a policy of inclusive education.

Inclusion takes two forms in French primary schools: 1) individual, where the child is supported in a regular class by a "School Life Assistant" (AVS), or 2) collective, in which children with disabilities are grouped in a specialised class and also spend times in their respective regular classes.

The Classes for School Inclusion (CLIS) are categorically defined by the disability and impairment: intellectual disabilities, hearing impairment, sight visual impairment and physical disabilities. CLIS is intended to support children with disabilities within their school, by providing teaching suited to individual needs. Specialist teachers have a maximum of twelve children aged between 6 and 12 years old in their care, with the mission of creating ideal learning situations for each one. A personalised schooling project (PPS) [1] organises the education for the child, who is expected to "attend, whenever possible, a regular class", commonly referred to as the "inclusion class". This attendance accounts for the inclusion time of these students. The CLIS 1, which, in 2010, represented 94% of specialised classes in primary school, (Delaubier, 2011, p.15), were specifically for children with for example a "disability stemming from cognitive or mental problems, including problems that inhibit development, such as challenges in language". (B.O. n° 31 du 27 août 2009).

This paper reports on the implementation of the inclusion of the children in CLIS 1, by means of research conducted in three specialised classes of three different French primary schools referred herein as CLIS Balzac, CLIS Baudelaire and CLIS Diderot. This doctoral study aimed to understand the experiences of these children in their school, from their voices. I will first clarify the different meanings of the concept of school inclusion, and describe the theoretical framework and methodology of my research. Finally, I will analyse the effects of the implementation of the inclusion policy in the three schools, for CLIS 1 children.

The different meanings of the concept

Scientific work regarding school inclusion has guided political decisions aiming to modify disabled children's educational situation. But what is the impact of these decisions on the meaning that professionals give to the term 'inclusion'?

The scientific meaning

Barton and Armstrong (2008) emphasise the relativity of the concept of inclusion in a world where competition between schools and countries constitutes a great obstacle to the development of inclusive education. "Against this background, notions such as "inclusion" and "human rights" must be seen as contingent, geographically and temporally situated concepts, rather than representing universal, shared values." (Barton, Armstrong, 2008, p.2). While school inclusion is a term well used in Canada and England, it has recently emerged in France (Kron, Plaisance, 2012). Unlike integration which demands that the child is accommodated to suit their environment, and in doing so 'erases their disability' (Stiker, 2005, p.158), inclusion requires alteration of the environment to suit the disabled child.

As such, inclusion it is inseparable from a democratic society, requiring "everyone's involvement in the collective well-being, and the incorporation of all in the different dimensions that underpin society" (Ebersold, 2009, p.73): each child, whoever he is, brings something to the group. Therefore, inclusion imposes on the school the expectation to consider itself, not solely as a place of knowledge transmission, but equally as a micro-society, where diversity is a key element of its organisation and working. Inclusion calls for the 'advent of the postnormative school" (Ebersold, 2009, p.74).

In demanding the best development of every child, inclusion redesigns the paradigm of the school: it is no longer possible to refer to a school norm, which demands that the students conform to the curriculum under the threat of being excluded from mainstream education.

In obliging the school system to adapt to the need's of individual children, inclusion requires teachers to rethink not only how they welcome these children, but also to critically reflect on the pedagogical approaches and the social experiences afforded the children in their school.

"Inclusive education is based on the prevention, elimination or reduction of the barriers of participation of all children"(Kron, Plaisance, 2012) It is, thus, an ethical response to difference. "Its aim is to respond, in the most equitable manner, to the diversity of students, so that all may find their place." (Zay, 2012, p.11) In this way, school inclusion is shown to be a political project that aims to develop an 'open democratic society' (Zay, 2012) by educating diverse children.

The political meaning

In France, the law of 11th February 2005 "for equal rights and opportunities, participation and citizenship of people with disabilities" aims to put into practice European recommendations regarding inclusive education. Disability is defined for the first time in an official text in terms of the consequences for the individual, rather than in terms of their deficiencies. This definition renders unconditional the principle right of each person with disabilities to fully exercise their citizenship. While this is consistent with the principles that underpin inclusion, the section of the law concerning the education of children with disabilities does not refer to explicitly to inclusion: inclusion is not yet a paradigm of disabled children's education.

As this law doesn't affect the status or operation of the CLIS, the acceptance of children is now up to the Departmental Home for Disabled people (MDPH), a unique public service that supports people with disabilities, and not National Education. [2] Whereas previously, National Education staff decided on the guidance of children, it is now the responsibility of a multidisciplinary team in which members of National Education are a minority. [3] This is a fundamental change as committee is formed of 23 members from different government sectors (e.g. political, administrative, medical-social, union, educational and other associations...). One third of the members represent people with disabilities and their families. This diversity aims to highlight the responsibility that the whole of society must take responsibility for these children. It is also acts an instrument of control over the school's proposed guidance of its children.

The circular of 17 July 2009, "Education of disabled children in primary school; updating of the organisation of School inclusion classes (CLIS)", specifies the provisions of the 2005 law. In this text, the CLIS are no longer school integration classes, but classes *for* school inclusion. The change in preposition is far from trivial. Inclusion is not designed as a fact, but as a process, a perspective. It therefore requires that procedures be established to achieve this goal. The circular advises that the education of children with disabilities is the concern of the pedagogical team, and not only the teacher in charge of the CLIS:

> *"The organisation and operation project of the CLIS involves all teachers in the school, in that one or two students of the CLIS may be enrolled in their class, at some point in time, depending on the teaching and learning goals which may vary considerably from one child to another. CLIS children are an integral part of organised activities for all children in the school project".* *(Circulaire n° 2009-087 du 17-7-2009)*

The word inclusion is mentioned only in the title of the circular, without further explanation, and the lexical precautions (each may be ... which can vary....) allow the circular to be interpreted differently, favouring diversity in its implementation, and without a clearly stated definition.

The professional meaning

In the school where the research was conducted, it was readily apparent that although placement in CLIS is officially the responsibility of the MDPH, it is the child's first school that typically determines this action, based on the academic performance of the child. The majority of the children who have participated in the research were placed in CLIS between the last year of nursery school and CE1 (cours élémentaire 1, age 7). This is consistent with the findings of Delaubier for the minister of National Education in 2011, "In many cases, it is the extent of the difficulties encountered in CP and CE1 which led to the referral to the CLIS, to identify the disability. (Delaubier, 2001, p.19). [4]

Delaubier highlights the impact of the law of 2005 on the inclusion of these children in regular classes:

> *"The same principle of acceptance by teachers in mainstream classes has progressed significantly in recent years. Times when a CLIS teacher is unable to find a child of his class access to one or two primary classes are rare." (Delaubier, 2011, p.27).*

But does the divided time in regular classes allow the children to form relationships with other children, does it make them feel part of a group, or does it isolate them from the school community? How are CLIS 1 children part of this undefined process?

Qualitative research

Participative research was conducted with children from three CLIS 1 classes of the greater Parisian region, in weekly class sessions of 40 minutes, and through participant observation time. In each class, the children developed a collective reflection about their place in the school, over ten sessions. The on-going development of allocated time spent in regular class, therapeutic and specific interventions, resulted in continual changes to the attendance of the children in CLIS. Twenty-eight of the 35 children enrolled in the three classes were observed, and participated in the study. The remaining children were absent during the research period.

Theoretical and methodological frameworks

According to René Lourau (1970), the institution is not defined solely in terms of organisational structures, but is dynamic where all of the actors play their part, and where there are power relations, personal and collective issues, emotional issues, and multiple contradictions. The research proposes to study these contradictions, based on analysers which are events occurring during research and shoving from the established rules. "The analyser is therefore both disruption and knowledge production" (Guillier, 2002, p.11) Here, different analysers were used to determine the effects of inclusion on the perceived place within the school of students from three CLIS 1: the words "handicap" and "inclusion", the ordinary classes' teachers, the inclusive practices. The implication, meaning « the libidinal relations, organizational and ideological which are developed between the subjects and the institutions." (Monceau, 2012, p.7) is crucial and is carefully analysed during this research. The institutional socio-clinic theorised by Monceau (2003), summarized these elements. It tries to understand the relations between the individuals, included the researcher, and the institutions by putting in place a collective disposal which explain them. This kind of research implies a real proximity of the researcher with the studied case. The researcher does not pose hypotheses, but rather must accept some uncertainty as the data are produced and analyzed. In this case, during the collective reflexion between the children of CLIS 1.

My research follows an epistemological and methodological framework that draws on the sociology of childhood, and which considers childhood to be a socially constructed idea, in which reality depends on the evolution of its society and the plans it defines for its people (Sirota, 2006). Childhood sociology views children as human beings rather than 'people in development'. Children are social actors, individually and collectively, within peer groups. In this context, the question we need to ask is "what does the child makes of his role" (Sirota, 2006, p.21). Through this research, the children were able to collectively share their reflections, despite sometimes obvious mechanistic barriers, including language. Consideration of these children from their collective reflections lead to the development of thought that produced usable data.

Collaborative research (Bourassa, 2012) should engage all of the participants in the field of practice. This study includes two distinct types of participants from the school world: teachers and children. If the teachers contributed to the analysis of the discourse of the children, to the development and constant evolution of the study, they affected the reflections very little, only taking authority when necessary, or reminding the children of an event. They developed the collective reflection autonomously, but the researcher suggested the subjects for discussion based on what activities were occurring at the time. Thus, I distinguish between the collaborative research carried out with the teachers and the participatory research with the children, by establishing a socio-clinical device. (Fablet, 2004, Monceau, 2012).

The socio-clinical device

Participative research was conducted with children in three stages: first, children took turns in photographing places in the classroom that they liked and disliked and then justified their choices in a second session. These photographs revealed various patterns which served as prompts for collective reflection in the second stage of the research. In two of the three classes, a final session was reserved for collaborative writing: one in the form of poster presentations with photographs, for the parents (at the request of the teacher), and in the other as an open letter to children in the rest of the school (as suggested by the children).

Reflection took place in three stages: 1) a collective review by the children of the previous session and the reading of the summary made by the researcher. This summary, validated or corrected collectively, assured the continuity of the reflexive process. Then I introduced the topic of discussion of the session. My interventions were limited to repeating remarks of students, to stimulate reflection when it was faltering, and/or to clarify what the children were saying. At the end of the session, I made an overall summary and announced the subject of the following session, defined in terms of their ideas for that day.

In all three classes, the photographs taken by the children revealed the importance of individual tables, mostly referred to as the 'favourite place' in the class. The first reflection was in this way part of this finding. Whatever the wording of the questions, and the reflective directions, children from the three classes addressed the same subjects, demonstrating similar concerns: differences between the CLIS and the regular classes, moving places in the school, relationships between them, relationships with adults and other children in the school, the question of difference and external intervention. However, the analysis of each class takes into account the diversity of inclusive practices in primary schools.

Analysis

The analysis was based on a comparative study of the discourse of the children in the three CLIS, teacher's comments, and my own observations. It was acquired in two steps: the syntheses were done during the collective research as the question of the implications expressed in my research agenda. These syntheses have identified different thematics which I have merged once the research finished in a first analysis. This analysis has exposed three main elements that I have developed. The dominance of the notion of teamwork has been studied from the reason of the presence of the children in a CLIS, from the choice of the photographs and their justification, from the perception of the children on the difference between the CLIS and ordinary classes. The question of the socialisation has been handled from the relations between the students of CLIS 1 and the other students of the school, the socialisation in the class, the identity building of the children of CLIS 1. The question of the inclusion has revealed the institutional responsibility at the macro-social level, its effects at micro-social level, the political responsibility on this question. This analysis helped to identify patterns, but also the differences revealing the issues of inclusion for these children.

Changing, evolving and multifaceted inclusions

Inclusion is individualised in different places and times: children may

133

be accommodated on a full or part time basis in CLIS. They share their time between school and a specialist establishment, or between school and home. Here, one child spends part of his/her time at home and three share their time between a day hospital and the CLIS. Another stopped her support in the day hospital. She then spent more time at school and stayed at home on Monday mornings. Four children are included full-time in a regular class. Due to this, they did not participate in the research. Their participation in CLIS is only administrative, but allows the MDPH to control their schooling. 26 children were in CLIS full-time. However, seventeen of them regularly leave the classroom for educational or therapeutic aid. Time and space are also divided within the school, as each child is required to know their inclusion times in the regular class.

Inclusions change depending on the projects of each class, external support, and the teacher who includes the student. Two children in the CLIS Balzac saw their inclusion times suspended, because their regular class teachers did not want them in their classes any longer. Two others, of the CLIS Diderot, only participated in the first three research sessions, because they were then included in physical education lessons in CP when I visited.

Inclusions are evolutional: The times spent in regular class is always evolving, depending on the progression or regression of children's educational results. Following two children's difficulties identified during their collective reflection sessions in CLIS Diderot, the teacher suspended their inclusion in their regular class for reading activities. One child from CLIS Balzac, having had his inclusion time increased, did not participate in the final sessions. One child from CLIS Baudelaire was included full time in CM2 (age 10, last year of primary school) during the research, especially following repeated requests stated during the collective reflection. *"Because I don't like this class; it embarrassed me that's all. I am with smallest and I don't like that."* (Charlene, CLIS Baudelaire).

Inclusions are multifaceted: they may be upon due to the school level of the child, their age, or both. One child may therefore be included in several regular classes, depending on the lesson. In this way, a child in the CLIS Diderot shared his time between four classes. The type of inclusion chosen is left to the discretion of the teachers, above all the CLIS teacher: they make individual contact with the teachers in whose regular class they wish a child to be included. In the three schools where I conducted my research, inclusions were not subject to collective pedagogical consultation, contrary to the recommendations of the 2009 circular.

In the CLIS Baudelaire and Diderot, teachers systematically included their children in one or more ordinary classes upon arrival to CLIS, whatever the child's school level or educational needs. Due to this, ten out of twenty-three children had one inclusion hour every day, in a class of an age group more than two years younger than them. Nine were included in a divided fashion, for artistic activities, physical education or reading classes. The teacher of the CLIS Balzac included only 4 children who she thought could follow the curriculum adapted to their age, minus a year or two [16]. Two children went to PE lessons in regular classes one hour per week, and four had no inclusion time.

Collective reflection

Collective reflection revealed three types of point of view, according to children's inclusion times.

Children who had no, or very little, inclusion times are satisfied with their place in the school and do not wish to change. *"CLIS is bringing me happiness"*, (Stefy, CLIS Balzac). Although they are the farthest from ordinary school life, they see themselves as *normal* students. This perception can be explained by the fact that they know only one class (The CLIS), by the individualisation of their learning and by their special situation with a specialist teacher (encouragement, value) that appears to provide them with a positive evaluation of their progress.

Children who have one daily hour of inclusion time for basic learning, are those that complained the most about their inclusions.

"There are things in the work of regular class, I can't do and, I do not like too well. The teacher is giving me some work but there are things that I don't understand." (Aziza, CLIS Diderot). They are always place with children who are younger than themselves, and they have experienced substantive learning challenges. Deviating from the school norm is thus the only time they are seen by the rest of the school. These children had contradictory responses: they wanted to return to regular classes with their same age peers and, at the same time, they wished to stop participating in inclusion times. Some also wanted collective inclusion times.

Children who have daily inclusion times (half or more of time at school) have already spent one or more years in CLIS. The gradual increase of their inclusion times is seen as a reward for their efforts and academic progress and allows them to see themselves like the other students. *"It is because I have well done my work; after my teacher told to the others classes that I was working well and so, I have been able to go in one of it."* (Fabien, CLIS Diderot). At the same time, they adapt the school norms and distinguish their times in the regular class, where they really learn, from the CLIS, where they rest. Recognition of the assistance provided by the class is accompanied by the gradual decrease of this class, over the years and increase of time in the normal class.

The discourse of the children about relationships with their peers were directly related to the inclusive practices of teachers. The children of CLIS Baudelaire and Diderot complained most about the other children in the school. *"Everybody is telling that we are disabled."* (Didier, CLIS Diderot). Their role, marked by their differences, by being part of a specialised class, is enhanced in the regular class by the visibility of their difficulties. In CLIS Balzac, children did not encounter major problems with the other children, because they were not identified in terms of disability. But in this class, 6 children had no or very little inclusion times. One may wonder whether the lack of explicit reference to the concept of inclusion in the 2009 circular has participated in the different implementations in the three CLIS studied.

The inclusion of children in CLIS 1

The differentiated discourse of the children regarding their experience of inclusion corresponded to the number of years they have spent in CLIS:

- Those who are satisfied to be there don't attend the regular classroom. Those who have been in CLIS for two years and spend half their school day in regular classes are also satisfied with this schooling arrangement.

- Those who complain have been in CLIS for at least a year, spend an hour every day in their regular classroom where they experience great difficulties, because they don't appear to have the academic capabilities required in this class.

In this example, CLIS fulfills its established mission for inclusive education. The inclusion process takes place in a cycle: where upon arrival, the child is not differentiated from his or her peers, then the child's differences are identified, and ultimately the child finds similarities with the students in the regular class where he or she spends half his school time.

The contradictions between the condemning of stigmatisation and isolation, and the assertion of children's well-being at school, brings us back to the notion of socialisation. In this case it is removed from discourse on the importance of schooling. Immersion in the normal school environment remains incomplete and generally has little impact in terms of peer socialization. Exchanges between CLIS children and regular class children are rare and when they do occur they are characterised by conflict. CLIS children keep to themselves, and even more so having spent several years in this class.

Conclusion

If the concept of inclusion is used from a lexical standpoint (i.e. how those at school use it), it is not yet consistent with its semantic dimension (i.e. the adaptation of the school to those with disabilities). In reality, the educational institution puts CLIS children in an integrative situation, rather than an inclusive one. Children are isolated from the rest of the school population, by fragmented inclusion times, which do not allow the creation of meaningful links with children in regular classes. The question of 'living together' that defines inclusion is not taken into account in the reality of the school. Inclusion is considered only in terms of individual learning, and not from a social standpoint.

As long as CLIS 1 children are kept in the school, their lack of academic capability will continue to separate them from ordinary school life. When they enter regular classes, the onus to adapt to the class is on them. In this class, if the teacher needs to individualise their learning, then they will be isolated from the rest of the group. Paradoxically, individualisation maintains an integrative logic, as it does not consider the child to be included in the group. We can therefore question the dialectic of this individualisation and this concept of inclusion.

Notes

[1] Various people are involved in the PPS: education professionals, health workers, and social service workers. It is signed by the parents.
[2] Departmental Home for Disabled People, responsible for the acceptance of disabled people, which has seven missions: "Information, acceptance and listening to disabled people, helping them plan their lives, assessing applications for Disability Compensation Benefit (PCH), guidance decisions, assuring the implementation of these decisions, support and mediation. ». http://www.senat.fr/rap/a11-109-6/a11-109-63.html

[3] CDAPH: Committee for the rights of the independence of disabled people, which informs the guidance decision of disabled children. See website http://www.social-sante.gouv.fr/informations-pratiques,89/fiches-pratiques,91/handicap-interlocuteurs-et,1898/la-commission-des-droits-et-de-l,12630.html

[4] French primary school, which serves children from 3 to eleven years old, is divided into three parts: Cycle 1, initial learning, in 1st, 2nd and 3rd year of preschool: Cycle 2, fundamental learning, in the preparatory class (CP), primary year one (CE1, age 7), primary year two (CE2, age 8): Cycle 3, consolidation learning, in middle year one (CM1, age 9) and middle year two (CM2, age 10). Official bulletin, September 5 2013.

References

Barton, L., & Armstrong, F. (2008). *Policy, experience and Change: Cross Cultural Reflexions on Inclusive Education*. London: Springer.

Bourassa, B., & Boudjaoui M., (dir.). (2012). *Des recherches collaboratives en sciences humaines et sociales*. Laval Canada: PUL.

Bulletin officiel de l'Education nationale n° 31 du 27 août 2009.

Bulletin officiel de l'Education nationale n° 32 du 5 septembre 2013.

Caraglio, M., & Delaubier, J.P. (2012). *La mise en œuvre de la loi du 11 février 2005 dans l'Education nationale*. Note n° 2012-100 juillet 2012. http://cache.media.education.gouv.fr/file/2012/95/7/2012-100_-_rapport_handicap_226957.pdf, retrieved January 16, 2014.

Circulaire n° 2009-087 du 17-7-2009 Scolarisation des élèves handicapés à l'école primaire; actualisation de l'organisation des classes pour l'inclusion scolaire (CLIS). *Bulletin officiel* n° 31, 27 août 2009.

Delaubier, J.P. (2012). *Les classes pour l'inclusion scolaire en 2010*. Note n° 2011-104 septembre 2011. http://media.education.gouv.fr/file/2011/53/8/2011-104-IGEN_215538.pdf, retrieved January 16, 2014.

Ebersold, S. (2009). Autour du mot inclusion, *Recherche et formation*, *61*, 71-83.

Fablet, D. (2004). Pour d'autres modalités de collaboration entre chercheurs et professionnels de l'intervention socio-éducative. *Éduquer* [En ligne], 8 | 2004, mis en ligne le 13 octobre 2008, consulté le 30 mars 2014. http://rechercheseducations.revues.org/345

Guillier, D. (2002). Petite histoire de l'analyseur argent. *Les Cahiers de l'implication. L'analyseur argent*, n° 5, hiver 01/02, 9-24.

Kron, M., & Plaisance, E. (2012). *Grandir ensemble, l'éducation inclusive dès la petite enfance.* Suresnes: INS HEA.

Loi n° 2005-102 du 11 février 2005 pour l'égalité des droits et des chances, la participation et la citoyenneté des personnes handicapées. *Journal Officiel de la République Française* n°36 du 12 février 2005 pp. 2353-2449.

Monceau, G. (dir.). (2012). *L'analyse institutionnelle des pratiques Une socio-clinique des tourments institutionnels au Brésil et en France.* Paris: L'Harmattan.

Projet de loi de finances pour 2012: solidarité, insertion et égalité des chances. http://www.senat.fr/rap/a11-109-6/a11-109-63.html, retrieved March 12, 2014

Sirota, R. (dir.). (2006). *Eléments pour une sociologie de l'enfance.* Rennes: PUR.

Stiker, H-J. (2005.) *Corps infirmes et sociétés.* Paris: Dunod. 3ème édition. 1ère édition, 1997, Paris: Aubier Montaigne.

Zay, D. (2012). *L'éducation inclusive. Une réponse à l'échec scolaire?* Préface de G. Langouët. Paris: l'Harmattan.

N° 14 | Octobre 2015

Recherches & Éducations

L'inclusion par l'éducation partagée

Dossier coordonné par
Joanne Deppeler & Danielle Zay

Revue de la Société Binet-Simon

RECHERCHES & EDUCATIONS

Dossier coordonné par Joanne Deppeler & Danielle Zay

N° 14 Octobre 2015

Ce numéro réunit des chercheurs œuvrant dans des milieux culturels très différents, Australie, Canada, Chine, Espagne, Etats-Unis, France, Grande-Bretagne, Taiwan, pour analyser les évolutions les plus récentes d'un principe orientant les politiques et pratiques des pays de l'OCDE : l'éducation inclusive.

En réponse aux critiques et contestations croissantes que suscite la mise en œuvre de réformes des systèmes éducatifs allant dans ce sens, les auteurs étudient l'évolution du concept à travers les recherches, les organisations internationales, les associations et les mouvements sociaux, les types d'organisation des systèmes scolaires et les pratiques des personnels d'éducation de tout ordre, enseignants, orthophonistes, psychologues, éducateurs spécialisés, etc., ainsi que les relations avec leurs partenaires, en particulier, les parents. À partir des résultats de ces recherches, sont analysés les défaillances, les dysfonctionnements et les solutions qui leur sont apportées dans différents pays et territoires.

À travers des études extrêmement diversifiées, se dégage l'idée, déjà exposée dans d'autres travaux sur d'autres thèmes, que, quelle qu'elle soit et, à quelque niveau que ce soit, la réussite scolaire et la prévention de l'échec sont une affaire de partage faisant une place à chaque catégorie d'acteurs sociaux qui en sont parties prenantes. Le jeu entre les forces sociales en présence et sa régulation restent, aujourd'hui comme hier, définis par la part à faire aux familles et aux professionnels, aux instances représentant le pouvoir central et les autorités locales. Ce qui est nouveau, c'est qu'on a beaucoup progressé dans deux voies : d'une part, l'idée que la complémentarité de partenaires divers peut seule apporter des réponses aux problèmes complexes d'une société diversifiée et de plus en plus hétérogène, d'autre part, dans les solutions à apporter aux problèmes inévitables que ces collaborations obligées suscitent. C'est ce dont ce numéro donne des exemples.

DOSSIER

■ **Editorial : L'éducation inclusive par l'éducation partagée**
Joanne Deppeler & Danielle Zay

■ **Education inclusive et changement social**
Danielle Zay

■ **Vers l'inclusion au-delà des murs de l'école :** *Un cas d'éducation inclusive contribuant à l'inclusion sociale en Espagne*
Lena de Botton, Ramón Flecha, Rocío García-Carrión, Silvia Molina

■ **Égalité et Qualité en éducation inclusive en Australie:** *Le cas des élèves en situation de handicap*
Joanne Deppeler, Chris Forlin, Dianne Chambers, Tim Loreman, Umesh Sharma

■ **Inclusion des étudiants malentendants dans les classes de langue étrangère:**
Récits d'expériences
Francois Victor Tochon & Yi-hung Liao

■ **Pratiques évaluatives des orthophonistes scolaires à l'égard des élèves de minorités culturelles : différenciation, uniformisation et normalisation**
Corina Borri-Anadon, Lorraine Savoie-Zajc, Monique Lebrun

■ **Les élèves des classes spécialisées de l'école élémentaire, entre intégration et inclusion**
Claire de Saint Martin

VARIA

■ **Patronymes médicaux des établissements scolaires parisiens :** *Un enjeu patrimonial ?*
Séverine Colinet

■ **Étude de l'impact d'une introduction des ateliers de philosophie dans les curriculums au primaire et au collège sur l'intégrité cognitive**
Bernard Slusarczyk, Gabriela Fiema, Aline Auriel, Emmanuèle Auriac-Slusarczyk

■ **Les hétérotopies, enjeux et rôles des espaces autres pour l'éducation et la formation** *Lieux collectifs et espaces personnels*
Emmanuel Nal

Bulletin d'abonnement

Recherches & Educations
Séverine Parayre
11 rue Charcot
92200 Neuilly sur Seine
recherches.et.educations@gmail.com

Société Binet-Simon

Nom................................Prénom......................................

Adresse..

Code postal..................Ville..

Pays..

Adresse électronique...

Commande de numéros : ....

Abonnements

☐ **Nouvel Abonnement Individuel** ☐ France 40 euros TTC ☐ (Dom-Tom) 44 euros TTC ☐ UE 50 euros TTC ☐ reste du monde 64 euros TTC

☐ **Réabonnement Individuel** ☐ France 34 euros TTC ☐ (Dom-Tom) 38 euros TTC ☐ UE 44 euros TTC ☐ reste du monde 60 euros TTC

☐ **Nouvel Abonnement étudiant et chômeur** ☐ France 34 euros TTC ☐ (Dom-Tom) 36 euros TTC ☐ UE 41 euros TTC ☐ reste du monde 55 euros TTC

☐ **Réabonnement étudiant et chômeur** ☐ France 30 euros TTC ☐ (Dom-Tom) 32 euros TTC ☐ UE 38 euros TCC ☐ reste du monde 51 euros TCC

☐ **Nouvel Abonnement Institution** ☐ France 54 euros TTC ☐ (Dom-Tom) 60 euros TTC ☐ UE 64 euros TTC ☐ reste du monde 79 euros TTC

☐ **Réabonnement Institution** ☐ France 50 euros TTC ☐ (Dom-Tom) 56 euros TTC ☐ UE 60 euros TTC ☐ reste du monde 75 euros TTC

Prix au numéro

☐ le numéro se commande via le site : i6doc.com

Avertissement :
Les numéros 1 à 6 ne sont plus disponibles en version papier. Ils sont désormais disponibles sur notre site internet. http://rechercheseducations.revues.org
Pour toutes commandes de tirages papiers, veuillez nous contacter à l'adresse suivante : recherches.et.educations@gmail.com

Chèque à l'ordre de la Société Binet-Simon

Date...

Signature..

Contributors to this Volume

Editors

Joanne Deppeler is Professor of Education and Associate Dean of Graduate Research in the Faculty of Education at Monash University, Victoria, Australia. She is committed to advancing theory, research and practice in the field of inclusive education and has had extensive experience in leading school development research projects focused on the professional learning of teachers within the context of improving inclusive practices. In particular, she is interested in finding new and innovative ways of researching the complexity of professional practice and learning in order to improve teacher quality and the outcomes of schooling for a range of students. For more than a decade she engaged in international inclusive education development and collaborative research (e.g. in Ukraine with Canadian partners, India, China and in Bangladesh and Ghana with doctoral students). Current research projects are focused on teacher education and equity and are in conjunction with a number of government funded research projects in Australia and in the South Pacific.

joanne.deppeler@monash.edu

Danielle Zay is Professor Emeritus at the University of Charles de Gaulle Lille 3. She graduated as an Economist from "Sciences Po" (Political Sciences), the IEP (Institute of Political Sciences) of Paris (France), ranked 5th worldwide in the 2015 QS World University rankings for Politics and International Studies. She began to work in private and public firms. She got the "agrégation" of philosophy (the highest selective exam to be recruited as a teacher) and chose teacher education and higher education. After passing her Ph.D. in Educational Sciences, she specialized in international projects and research on cross-institutional partnerships, in particular to deal with youth at risk. Her projects were supported by the European Commission and the ERDF (European Regional Development Fund). She created and was the "Main Convenor" of the European Educational Research Association (EERA) Network 15, "Research Partnerships in Education" (1998-2007). Her numerous publications have appeared in French, English and Spanish. She is the Book Series Editor of *Inclusive Education and Partnerships*, Deep University Press. *zaydanielle@gmail.com*

Other Contributors

Corina Borri-Anadon teaches in the Education Department at the University of Quebec in Trois-Rivières, Canada. She holds a Master's degree in speech therapy and has completed a Ph.D. in education at the University of Quebec in Montreal analyzing assessment practices of school speech therapists working with cultural minority students. She's a regular member of the Laboratoire sur l'inclusion scolaire (LISIS) and the Centre d'études ethniques des universités montréalaises (CEETUM) and co-director of the *Observatoire sur la formation à la diversité et l'équité* (www.ofde.ca). Her academic work overlaps both special education and ethnic relations in education fields. It focuses on 3 main axis: ethno-cultural, linguistic and religious diversity in training school personnel, inclusion-exclusion issues in special education and paramedical personnel practices in schools.
Corina.Borri-Anadon@uqtr.ca

Lena de Botton is Lecturer of Sociology, in the Department of Sociological Theory, Philosophy of Law and Methodology of Social Sciences at the University of Barcelona, Spain. She obtained her PhD at the École des Hautes Études en Sciences Sociales – EHESS Paris. Her research interests combine education and sociology and evolve

around multiculturalism; dialogic feminism, including women across cultures; migrations; and interreligious dialogue.
lenadebotton@ub.edu

Dianne Chambers is Associate Professor in the School of Education at the University of Notre Dame, Australia. Her research in inclusive education is focused on pre-service teacher education, resource allocation for schools, and information technology to support student diversity.
dianne.chambers1@nd.edu.au

Ramón Flecha is Professor of Sociology in the Department of Sociological Theory, Philosophy of Law and Methodology of Social Sciences at the University of Barcelona, Spain. He is currently directing the EU-funded research IMPACT-EV (FP7, European Commission), which aims at developing indicators and standards that will serve to evaluate not only the scientific impact of research in Social Sciences and Humanities, but particularly its political and social impact. He also directed the INCLUD-ED project, the only one in social sciences included among the 10 successful scientific investigations published by the European Commission.
ramon.flecha@ub.edu

Chris Forlin, previously Professor at Honk Kong Institute of Education, now works as an international education consultant specialising in inclusive education research and consultancies with government and universities.
chrisforlin@outlook.com

Rocío García-Carrión is Marie Curie Postdoctoral Research Fellow at the University of Cambridge, Faculty of Education and Research

Associate at Wolfson College, Cambridge, UK. She is leading the FP7 EU-funded project ChiPE, aiming at developing inclusive epistemic climates in primary schools. Her research conducted at CREA included dialogic learning, classroom interaction, schools as learning communities, educational inclusion of Roma children and excluded populations in urban schools.
rgc31@cam.ac.uk

Monique Lebrun is Professor Emeritus from the University of Quebec in Montreal, Canada. She has conducted research in language teaching for thirty years and is the author of over 200 scientific papers and of a dozen books about reading, literature teaching and digital literacy. She was vice president of the International Federation of Teachers of French and was awarded by France the title of Knight of Arts and Letters.
lebrun-brossard.monique@uqam.ca

Yi-Hung Liao is Assistant Professor in the Department of English at Wenzao Ursuline University of Languages in Kaohsiung, Taiwan, R.O.C. She is an alumni from the University of Wisconsin where she did her doctoral studies. Her research interests include transnational inquiries of curriculum planning and postmodern approaches of inclusive education.
99290@mail.wzu.edu.tw

Tim Loreman is Professor of Education and Associate Vice President Academic at Concordia University of Edmonton in Canada. His research interests include inclusive education, teacher education, and pedagogy.
tim.loreman@concordia.ab.ca

Silvia Molina is Adjunct Professor at the Department of Pedagogy, Faculty of Education and Psychology at the University Rovira i Virgili, Tarragona, Spain. Her research interests evolve around inclusive education, education of students with disabilities and learning communities.
silvia.molina@urv.cat

Claire de Saint Martin works at the Université de Cergy Pontoise, France (Laboratoire Education, Mutations, Apprentissages). She is a special educator working with children with cognitive disabilities and with pervasive developmental disorder. Current research uses students' voices to understand their perceptions about their place in school, with the concept of liminality as defined by Robert F. Murphy as starting point. Her research and teaching interests focus on concept of liminality, concept of inclusion, schooling of children with disabilities, sociology of childhood, scientist-practitioner model, institutional analysis, methodologies of qualitative research, Institutional socio-clinic.
clairesm1709@hotmail.fr

Lorraine Savoie-Zajc is Professor Emeritus from the School of Education, University of Quebec in Outaouais, Gatineau, Quebec, Canada. She has conducted researches dealing with the processes of change in education and more specifically addressing school teachers' and directors' professional development. She is currently involved in researches using learning communities as a means to support teachers in the adjustment of professional practices.
lorraine.savoie@uqo.ca

Umesh Sharma is Associate Professor in the Faculty of Education at Monash University, Victoria, Australia. His international inclusive education research has been developed in partnerships in Canada,

USA, UK, in several Asian contexts, South Africa, Brunei and Brazil and most recently in island countries of the South Pacific. *umesh.sharma@monash.edu*

François Victor Tochon is Professor of Curriculum & Instruction (School of Education) and French Education (Department of French and Italian) at the University of Wisconsin-Madison, Madison, USA. He proposes a deep, inclusive approach to Curriculum, Pedagogy & Education to end collective self-destructive behavior through shared understanding emerging from cross-cultural dialogue. Hearing impaired people represent another culture we should learn. *ftochon@education.wisc.edu*

Deep University Online !

For updates and more resources

Visit the Deep University Website:

www.deepuniversity.net

deepuniversitypress.org

Contact: publisher@deepuniversity.net

❖ Facebook group on Deep Language Learning:
https://www.facebook.com/groups/deep.approach/

❖ Twitter: http://twitter.com/Deep_Approach

http://www.languageeducationpolicy.org

Correspondence for this volume

Danielle Zay

zaydanielle@gmail.com

Dr. Manuel Fernandez Cruz, Prof., University of Granada, Spain

Dr. Stephanie Fonvielle, Associate Prof., Teacher Education University Institute, University of Aix-Marseille, France

Dr. Elliot Gaines, Prof., Wright State University, President of the Semiotic Society of America, Internat. Communicology Institute

Dr. Mingle Gao, Dean, College of Education, Beijing Language and Culture University (BLCU), Beijing, China

Dr. Mercedes González Sanmamed, Prof. University of Coruña, Spain

Dr. Gabriela Hernández Vega, Prof., University of Nariño, Colombia

Dr. Xiang Long, Guilin University of Electronic Technology, China

Dr. Maria Masucci, Drew University, New Jersey, USA

Dr. Liliana Morandi, Associate Prof., National University of Rio Cuarto, Cordoba, Argentina

Dr. Joëlle Morrissette, Prof., Department of Educational Psychology, Université of Montreal, Quebec, Canada

Dr. Martha Murzi Vivas, Prof., University of Los Andes, Venezuela

Dr. Thi Cuc Phuong Nguyen, Vice Rector, Hanoi University, Vietnam

Dr. Shirley O'Neill, Associate Prof., President of the International Society for leadership in Pedagogies and Learning, University of Southern Queensland, Australia

Dr. José-Luis Ortega, Prof., Foreign Language Education, Faculty of Education, University of Granada, Spain

Dr. Surendra Pathak, Head and Prof., Department of Value Education, IASE University of Gandhi Viday Mandir, India

Dr. Charls Pearson, Logic, Semiotics, Philosophy of Science, Peirce Studies, Director of Research, Semiotics Research Institute

Dr. Luis Porta Vázquez, Prof. at the National University of Mar del Plata CONICET (Argentina)

Inclusive Education and Partnerships Book Series

Dr. Danielle Zay, Book Series Editor
Professor Emeritus, University of Charles de Gaulle Lille 3, France

This collection aims at developing an in-depth understanding of inclusive education as well as its related practices. Inclusive education main principle is anchored in the right to education each citizen, coming from democratic societies, is endowed with. This person can develop to its full potential and live a better life. Biological, psychological, cultural, racial, social differences are not seen as problems meant to exclude but as resources and a wealth for the living together. Inclusive education is conceived so to emphasize the notions of sharing and partnerships. Sharing of ideas, sharing of research results, sharing of practices from partners coming from various fields and various perspectives, all those are seen as most helpful in the understanding of inclusion linked problems, thanks to a systemic perspective. Such a rich understanding will encourage the emergence of innovative solutions most susceptible to adequately meet growingly complex and technologically advanced societies needs.

The collection welcomes researches dealing with learners whose visible or invisible differences are seen and treated as handicaps as well as researches focused upon educational policies, resources and practices dealing with inclusive education. The collection seeks also to publish articles dealing with normalization issues educational systems cope with in order to answer work-related needs in a global market world. It is reaffirmed that each learner' capacities are not equally taken into account with the curriculum structure and with learning methods when it is uniformly applied to all. In this regards, partnerships among social actors, users (learners, families), practitioners, educators and professionals from fields such as education, health, culture and from associative organisms are seen as bearers of innovative and effective solutions.

www.deepuniversitypress.org/inclusive-education-and-partnerships.html

Deep Language Learning
Book Series

François Victor Tochon, Prof., University of Wisconsin-Madison
Shirley O'Neill, Assoc. Prof., University of Southern Queensland, Au
Zuleyha Colak, Assistant Prof., Columbia University
Xiang Long, Assist. Dean/Chair of the Institute of Foreign Language
General Education, Guilin U. of Electronic Technology, China
Jianfang Xiao, Assoc. Prof., School of English and Education
Guangdong University of Foreign Studies, Canton, China

Book editor and advisory editorial board members

Language learning needs to be reconceptualized in two ways: first, as an expression of dynamic planning prototypes that can be activated through self-directed projects. Second, integrating structure and agency to meet deeper, humane aims. The dynamism of human exchange is meaning- producing through multiple connected intentions among language task domains.

Language-learning tasks have a cross-cultural purpose which then become meaningful within broader projects that meet higher values and aims such as deep ecology, deep culture, deep politics and deep humane economics. Applied semiotics will be a tool beyond the linguistic in favor of value-loaded projects that are chosen in order to revolutionize the current state of affairs, in increasing our sense of responsibility for our actions as humans vis-à-vis our fellow humans and our home planet. In this respect, deep instructional planning offers a grammar for action. Understanding adaptive and complex cross-cultural situations is the prime focus of such a hermeneutic inquiry.

For more, see here:

http://deepuniversitypress.org/deep-language-learning.html

Language Education Policy
Book Series

Language Education Policy (LEP) is the process through which the ideals, goals, and contents of a language policy can be realized in education practices. Language policies express ideological processes. Their analysis reveals the perceptions of realities proper to certain sociocultural contexts. LEPs further their ideologies by defining and disseminating the values of policymakers. Because Language Education Policies are related to status, ideology, and vision of what society should be and traditions of thoughts, such issues are complex, quickly evolving, submitted to trends and political views, and they need to be studied calmly. The way to approach them is to get comparative information on what has been done in many settings, which are working or not, which are their flaws and merits, and try to grasp the contextual variables that might apply in specific locations, without generalizing too fast.

Policy discourses and curricula reveal the ideological framing of the constructs that they encode and create, project, enact, and enforce aspects such as language status, power and rights through projective texts generated to forward and describe the contexts of their enactments. Policy documents are therefore socially transformative through their evaluative function that frames and guides action in order to achieve language reforms. While temperance and reflection are required to address such complex issues, because moving to fast may create trouble, nonetheless the absence of action in this domain may lead to systemic intolerance, injustice, inequity, mass discrimination and even, genocidal crimes.

http://www.deepuniversitypress.org/language-education-policy.html

http://www.languageeducationpolicy.org

Deep Activism
Book Series

Dr. Araceli Alonso, Associate Faculty
University of Wisconsin-Madison
Dr. Langle de Paz, Founder & co-director Foundation for a Culture
of Peace, and researcher of the Institute for Human Rights,
Democracy and Culture of Peace and Non-Violence at the
Autonomous University of Madrid

Book Editors

Deep politics could challenge the status quo. Examining everyday politics and reconceptualizing the position of the citizen, consider that acting on social representations might help the change process to address social hierarchies and inequalities. Our institutional systems do not tolerate critical examination but rather support conformity, norms, standards and obedience. The goal of a deep activism is to "removing ourselves from mental slavery…and enter into a humanist inquiry project that employs imagination to foster change" (Andrew Gitlin, p.22, in the Educational Researcher). Everyday politic is grounded in ruled relations, it shapes "how we see people, our relations with those different from ourselves, and the conclusions that we draw about those relationships" (p.15). Deep activism, rather than focusing on resisting the reproduction of hierarchies, centers on a freedom quest. It uses "imagination to redefine normative categories" (p.16), thereby initiating a process that can create a new terrain for equality. Thus deep activism links aesthetics with inquiry as a living process. Its commitment to social justice manifests through aesthetics to envision and create alternative imaginaries.

http://www.deepuniversitypress.org/deep-activism.html

Deep Education
Book Series

François Victor Tochon, Prof., University of Wisconsin-Madison
Zuleyha Colak, Assistant Prof., Columbia University
Deming Mei, Dean, College of International Programs, Shanghai
International Studies University
Shirley O'Neill, Prof., University of Southern Queensland, Australia

Book editor and advisory editorial board members

The concept of "depth" in education emerged from a variety of disciplines, with the recognition that continuing business as usual didn't make sense within the current state of affaires in Education. Current shallow teaching and learning practices need to be interrupted. New formats should be explored for Education at large. There are certainly new, more profound ways of understanding each discipline, and teaching and learning them. Disciplinary fields such as philosophy and educational philosophy, ecology, economy, cultural studies, psychology, ecopsychology and educational psychology have gone through a drastic revision of their curriculum approaches—not to speak of various other disciplines—in terms of depth of knowledge and deep reading (Roberts & Roberts, 2008). The time is ripe to introduce a new approach to Education.

For more, see

http://www.deepuniversitypress.org/deep-education.html

Help Them Learn a Language Deeply

Dr. François Victor Tochon
University of Wisconsin-Madison

The advocates for an effective U.S. policy for teaching and learning world languages could benefit from reading this critical contribution. Tochon's conceptualization of a "deep approach" is both timely and profoundly better for preparing learners for the globally interconnected realities they live now. Tochon provides viable options that show authentic language learning is profoundly connected to shaping thinking and social actions, as well as to further language and literacy learning. No longer can world language education be confined to merely a show of empty linguistic performances, rather needs to directed more towards building performances that truly put language to work on addressing sociocultural realities, forging ahead in the spirit of Dewey, Vygotsky, & Freire. —*Theresa Austin, Professor, Author of "Content-Based Second Language Teaching and Learning", School of Education, University of Massachusetts, Amherst*

Tochon's conceptualization of the deep approach to the study of world languages, unlike most changes in foreign language education, is not simply a change in approach or methodology. It is far more fundamental than this – it is, indeed, a paradigm shift, that requires us to rethink virtually everything that we assume about the teaching and learning of languages. It is also one of the most exciting, creative and powerful ideas to emerge in our field in decades, and creates incredible opportunities for all of us. —*Timothy Reagan, Author of "Language, Education, and Ideology" and "The Foreign Language Educator in Society" (with T. Osborn), Professor and Dean of the College of Education and Human Development at the University of Maine in Orono*

For more see

http://www.deepuniversitypress.org/help.html

Language Education Policy Unlimited: Global Perspectives and Local Practices

Dr. François Victor Tochon, Editor
University of Wisconsin-Madison

"This essential book shows why language education policy will never work if it is top-down and ignores local contexts and stakeholders. It illustrates the fundamental importance of taking local contexts into consideration and actively engaging and empowering local stakeholders in the development and implementation of all language education policy. A better blueprint for successful language education policy would be hard to find." — *Dr. Andy Kirkpatrick, Griffith University, Australia*

This book is a first. Language Education Policy is a new field of study that establishes a cross section between educational policy and language policy studies. It inherits from an abundance of intellectual and methodological traditions while opening new perspectives that focus on the interface between policymaking and its enactment in a classroom or an educational setting. The study of the interface between the macro-policy level of the political stage and the micro-policies of education in practice implies a focus on how policy decisions are translated into regulations that affect the lives of people. 21 authors have contributed to this outstanding volume that situates the stakes in the new field of inquiry with examples in 14 countries.

http://www.deepuniversitypress.org/lep.html

FROM TRANSNATIONAL LANGUAGE POLICY TRANSFER TO LOCAL APPROPRIATION
The case of the National Bilingual Program in Medellín, Colombia

Dr. Jaime Usma Wilches

University of Antioquia

Drawing on the example of Medellín, Colombia, Jaime Usma's book does a magnificent work at dismantling one of the most pervasive grand narratives in globalized transnational foreign language policies: proficiency in English as one of the strongest pillars of a vibrant modern knowledge society, associated with higher economic gains for all. The author cogently demonstrates how apparently neutral and technically sound transnational and national policymaking fails to properly address structural inequality and social and economic injustice, while being creatively reenacted by local schools and actors that appropriate them according to their own goals, needs, and desires towards a more just and humane society.

—*Maria Alfredo Moreira, University of Minho, Portugal*

World wide there is a growing awareness that properly explanatory accounts of language education policy must fuse national and local perspectives, questions of structure and argument, evidence and debate and of course the various interests of the diverse players involved.

Dr Jaime Usma has made a notable contribution to this more sophisticated approach to LP with this excellent and internationally relevant analysis of Colombia's national government policy, the appropriation/adaptation of central policy in the city of Medellín and the views, experiences and accounts of teachers, officials, experts and communities and transnational agencies. In addition to its LP relevance the book has much to say about how English is constituted in an increasing number of settings globally and how claims and counterclaims about global English resonate at different levels and among different interests. All in all an excellent and worthwhile volume. —*Joseph Lo Bianco, Professor of Language and Literacy Education, The University of Melbourne, Australia*

http://www.deepuniversitypress.org/medellin.html

162

Guide to Authors

What our Publishing Team can offer:

➤ An international editorial team, in more than 20 universities around the world.

➤ Dedicated and experienced topic editors who will review and provide feedback on your initial proposal.

➤ A specific format that will speed up the production of your book and its publication.

➤ Higher royalties than most publishers and a discount on batch orders.

➤ Global distribution and marketing in the U.S., UK, Europe, Australia, Brazil, China, Mexico, Russia, and Asian countries.

➤ Fair recognition of your work in your area of specialization.

➤ Quality design and affordable sales pricing. Using the latest technology, our books are produced efficiently, quickly and attractively.

➤ A global marketing plan, including electronic and web marketing on social networks and review mailing.

http://deepuniversitypress.org

➤ Contact: publisher@deepuniversity.net

www.ingramcontent.com/pod-product-compliance
Lightning Source LLC
Chambersburg PA
CBHW050526270326
41926CB00015B/3093